Demystifying
American Yoga

ALSO BY SARAH HENTGES
AND FROM MCFARLAND

*Teaching Girls on Fire: Essays on Dystopian
Young Adult Literature in the Classroom*
(edited by Sarah Hentges and Sean P. Connors, 2020)

*Girls on Fire: Transformative Heroines
in Young Adult Dystopian Literature* (2018)

Women and Fitness in American Culture (2014)

*Pictures of Girlhood:
Modern Female Adolescence on Film* (2006)

Demystifying American Yoga

Embodied Movement for Individual and Collective Transformation

Sarah Hentges

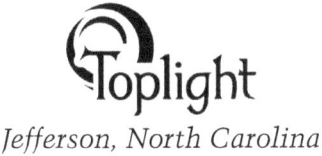

Jefferson, North Carolina

LIBRARY OF CONGRESS CATALOGING-IN-PUBLICATION DATA

Names: Hentges, Sarah, 1976– author.
Title: Demystifying American yoga : embodied movement for individual and collective transformation / Sarah Hentges.
Description: Jefferson, North Carolina : Toplight, 2025 | Includes bibliographical references and index.
Identifiers: LCCN 2024057122 | ISBN 9781476695679 (paperback : acid free paper) ∞
 ISBN 9781476655406 (ebook)
Subjects: LCSH: Yoga. | Physical fitness for women—United States—Social aspects.
Classification: LCC B132.Y6 H377 2025 | DDC 181/.450973—dc23/eng/20241228
LC record available at https://lccn.loc.gov/2024057122

ISBN (print) 978-1-4766-9567-9
ISBN (ebook) 978-1-4766-5540-6

© 2025 Sarah Hentges. All rights reserved

No part of this book may be reproduced or transmitted in any form or by any means, electronic or mechanical, including photocopying or recording, or by any information storage and retrieval system, without permission in writing from the publisher.

Printed in the United States of America

Toplight is an imprint of McFarland & Company, Inc., Publishers

*Box 611, Jefferson, North Carolina 28640
www.toplightbooks.com*

To the students
in my overlapping communities

"Practice is how we become what we long to be."
—adrienne maree brown, *Holding Change*

"This is all practice, not just for ourselves but for the seeds that will float out from our struggles—and our calmness—to help feed whatever comes next."
—Susan Raffo, *Liberated to the Bone*

"Engaging in the practices that bring up some discomfort—and coming into contact with our *edge*—is often where we find the most nourishing metaphorical juice for our healing needs."
—Jamie Marich, *Process Not Perfection*

"But yoga isn't supposed to feel good or comfortable. It's about understanding what it *means* to be uncomfortable. No one is exempt from the rough edges. The further you go, the uglier it gets. But that can't be a reason to avoid the work."
—Jessamyn Stanley, *Yoke: My Yoga of Self-Acceptance*

"To lead a practice of social justice through yoga one must make a commitment to revisit and recommit to love again and again."
—Michelle Cassandra Johnson, *Skill in Action*

Table of Contents

Gratitude	ix
Deconstructed Land Acknowledgment and Invocation	xii
Preface	1
Interlude: Building the Toolbox	4
Introduction	7
Interlude: Just Breathe	20
ONE. Discover and Practice	29
Interlude: Exploring Your Self and Embracing the "Woo-Woo"	51
TWO. Unpack	66
Interlude: Yoga Tools Off the Mat	123
THREE. Imagine	144
FOUR. Play	199
Conclusions	233
EXPAND (Works Cited)	237
Index	243

Gratitude

I am grateful for all that I am.
I am thankful for all that I have.
I am humbled by all that I know.
I am humbled by all that I don't know.
I am grateful for the opportunity for more life,
   more love, more peace, more connection.
I am.

Most books have an acknowledgments section, but since this is a book about yoga, I have chosen to approach this aspect through the lens of gratitude—a cornerstone to yoga and mindfulness. When we are grateful, we are able to appreciate what we have instead of obsessing over what we don't have. Americans love to obsess about what we don't have, what we want, what we think we deserve. Letting go of this obsession is one kind of transformation.

I am grateful for every resource that informs this book, and I pay homage to the writers, thinkers, and practitioners throughout this book, as well as in the "Play" section. I am grateful for YogaFit Worldwide Training Systems, founded by Beth Shaw, where I discovered yoga at my first training in 2005. And for JourneyDance, created by Toni Bergins and facilitated by Joan White-Hansen and Joy Okoye, which brought my yoga explorations together with my love for dance and has helped me create embodied movement offerings that were trying to emerge. JourneyDance has been full of synchronicities and made me way more woo-woo than I ever could have imagined. Both of these training programs have empowered me and connected me with community beyond the local. And we are all helping to make the world a better place. I am also grateful for Elise Boynton and Sea

Change Yoga for providing a model of socially conscious, healing yoga and connecting me to a not-quite-local community.

I am grateful for my local community/my daily reality—my friends, colleagues, students, collaborators, participants. This community continues to grow through The Spiral Goddess Collective and I am grateful for Lisa Black, Gwyn Estey-Kendall, Kati Corlew, Betty McCue-Herlihy, Suzanne Kelly and so many more who have been friends and colleagues as well as participants in my classes and workshops. Karyssa Murchison, Alex Gilgan, Trish Hanley-Goodwin, Christine Little, and Lisa Taplin-Murray supported this dream from the start. We will circle back. I am grateful for Rori Knott, for her mental health therapy that helped to pull me out of despair and put me on a path toward healing—and for her Rest, Restore, Renew yoga mini-retreats that I never miss. I am beyond grateful for Sen Wilde and Kate Mikkelsen who have helped to support and grow this collective, taking on so much of what I just can't manage, and bringing their talents and gifts to our collective community.

I am grateful to all of my students, especially those in my Integrative Yoga and Embodied Social Justice classes. I wish I could name them all here. As I tell anyone who will listen, my students are brilliant. I am humbled to create opportunities for them to grow and unfurl their influence into the world. Their insight and passion have fueled my soul while their struggles have broken my heart and reinforced my drive to continue my work in and out of academia. I am endlessly grateful to Rachel Larrivee, my student and teaching assistant, editor and more. I will be waiting for the opportunity to help her birth her book into the world.

Years ago, Tessa Pyles, my former student turned closest friend, read a very early and very different version of this book. I'm hoping this version will help to inspire her to move her body, heal her trauma, and care for herself like never before. I am grateful for her unconditional love and support throughout the years. And for the comradery, support, and collaboration with my fitness soul sister, Kristy McNaughton. She brings her own brand of this magic to her community. I am grateful for Heidi Niles and her support as well as for my former YMCA fitness family—I am the radical outcast that played their game as long as I could. Their support over the years helped me to get to where I am today.

And, finally, I am grateful for my mother, Nancy Monroe, who planted seeds of dance (and creativity and writing and feminism and more) early in my life and has been my biggest supporter, even when I am critical of what she gave me and maybe forget to be as grateful as I should be.

I am grateful for everyone who does the work (within and without) to create a more embodied, connected, inclusive, loving, and just world where we can all breathe and grow, heal and transform.

Deconstructed Land Acknowledgment and Invocation

> "We are volcanoes. When we women offer our experience as our truth, as human truth, all the maps change. There are new mountains."
> —Ursula LeGuin

We stand like mountains. Grounded, powerful, slightly shifting.

We inhale radical self-love from our heart down through our belly, down through our legs, down through our toes, down through our roots. Letting our roots run deep, letting them spread out like a mycelium network, nourishing trees and plants and sustaining life.

As Sonya Renee Taylor reminds us, "If radical self-love is an oak tree, it is an essential part of an entire ecosystem. When it grows stronger, the entire system does as well" (2–3).

We exhale love through our roots and tap into the long lineage and evolution of yoga, from ancient India and, wider, North Africa, and wider, from indigenous peoples and traditions in the Americas and around the world. We honor these sacred roots and our shared ecosystem with our recognition and love.

We inhale up through our roots as we recognize the land where we live, love, breathe, work, and find community, acknowledging that here in the U.S. what we have was built on stolen land and by forced labor. We pay back this debt by keeping our eyes, ears, minds, and hearts open and settling for nothing less than justice, equity, peace, and love.

We remember Taylor's words: "Radical self-love demands that

we see ourselves and others in the fullness of our complexities and intersections and that we work to create space for those intersections" (9).

As we breathe together, our hearts are connected; we intersect across time and space. We let our breath be as abundant as our love—as expansive. Our love reaches up and out into everything bigger than we are, everything that is bigger than we can know or understand.

Our love expands into the infinite possibility of the universe, finding space for growth, for transformation. And that love returns right here, to where we stand together. Through our love, we take a stand.

Inhaling—sending self-love, *radical* self-love throughout our bodies.

Exhaling—sending love out into the space around us, the world around us.

Strong. Stable. Grounded. Humble. Interconnected.

We are new mountains.

Preface

Sit on your organic rye-stuffed meditation cushion. Close your eyes and breathe until you find enlightenment. Reach down and adjust your over-priced yoga pants while you chant "Om." Mentally make your shopping list. Wonder why the woman next to you is breathing so loudly. Get frustrated when your body won't do what *that* body over there does with ease and grace. Chuckle at the yoga puns that adorn the tank tops all around you. Roll your eyes when the woman at the front of the classroom busts into a spontaneous handstand. Berate yourself for not being in the moment. Are you doing yoga yet?

You hear about it everywhere. You see it in commercials, in movies, on television, and all over social media. Your co-worker goes there after work. Your doctor told you to try some yoga for your low back pain. Your neighbor's grandmother meditates. The local strip mall has a hot yoga studio. Your kids do yoga instead of detention. You wonder: what's all the *hype* about *stretching*?

You tried it once or twice. Or, you take a few classes per week. Or, you've always wanted to try it. You fear it. It's boring, too slow, and it doesn't burn enough calories; or, it's a blasphemous activity. You don't have a yoga mat; you don't have a yoga butt.

Or, you are totally committed to the transformative life experience that yoga has been for you. You've attended a retreat in Bali and a workshop at the Yoga Journal LIVE! conference. Or, you took a 200-hour training through a yoga school and registered with Yoga Alliance. Maybe you keep meaning to get back to it. Maybe you don't know where to begin.

Regardless of where your yoga journey began, where it is now, or where you may have gone with it, yoga can always be experienced in new ways. Yoga can be shaken loose. It can shake us loose and put us back together.

Regardless of where we are on the life-long journey that is yoga, we can all take a little something—or a lot of something—away from this book. Some things may sound ridiculously simple, incredibly silly, helplessly romantic, optimistically misguided, deceptively easy, uncompromisingly idealistic but, ultimately, new insights—however large and life-changing or small and seemingly insignificant—are what this book is about. Creative/critical insights for the mind and the body. Creative/critical insights for considering ourselves and the world around us.

This book is not indulgent self-help. This book isn't an exercise manual or a diet plan. It does not provide detailed instruction or attempt to bend you into uncomfortable postures, though it may bend you into uncomfortable thought experiences. It will not make you thinner or younger or more beautiful or a better person. This book will not, on its own, provide a spiritual awakening; nor will it teach you how to navigate the pressures of our complex world. This book is an opportunity. It is an invitation to step outside the box and it encourages unfettered, embodied, emboldened exploration.

This book is also a reminder that learning is often uncomfortable. Thus, *Demystifying American Yoga* asks us to consider what yoga means to people in a variety of (literal and figurative) places with different goals and experiences. However, this book is not an attempt to catalog the philosophies, practices, and meanings. It does not roll out a long linear history or attempt to be exhaustive. You will only occasionally find me dropping *Sanskrit* (the traditional language of yoga), but not in an attempt to appear authentic. I do not attempt to be fair and balanced. Instead, we'll consider the various uses of this yoga tool—the ways it is abused and exploited by capitalism and white supremacy; the ways it can be used as a means of disassociating and avoiding difficult feelings and conversations; the ways it can be robbed of deeper meaning through cultural appropriation and spiritual bypassing; the ways it can be manipulated and unleashed by those with power, privilege, and influence upon the vulnerable, ignorant or innocent.

But we'll also look at the ways in which yoga can be enlightening, expanding, earth-shattering, and empowering. We'll explore the ways in which people's lives are transformed, the ways in which yoga heals physical and mental wounds, and the ways in which a lens of yoga can be used to challenge and re-make outmoded, ineffective institutions. We'll see yoga as a personal practice and as a cultural phenomenon, as well as a pool of transformative potential we have only begun to tap.

What *Demystifying American Yoga* aims for is space—in your head and in your body—space that you can keep for yourself or share with other people, space you can lounge and languish in, space you can take up, space that you think and move in, space that provides opportunities to grow. But no pressure. There are no miracles here, only hard work. Only letting go. Only pleasure. The work is a life-long process with ups and downs, ebb and flow. The possibilities are limitless, unbound and unbinding. Don't be too scared.

Simply put, I want to explore, expand, and unpack American yoga in all of its incarnations and applications—as it has been sold, packaged, practiced, offered, applied, imagined, and reimagined. Through critical and creative explorations, I want to simultaneously complicate and simplify yoga, to give us new ways of thinking about our minds and bodies and about spirituality. I aim to share techniques that can have powerful practical benefits, and to provide a space for creativity and innovation that is grounded in reality and prepares us for an ever-evolving, increasingly complex world. Yoga is only a tool. We decide how to use it. This unconventional yoga book only asks that you move and be moved. We may lose ourselves and find ourselves many times, but the mind/body/spirit practices of yoga bring us back to ourselves and to each other again and again. By demystifying and re-envisioning American yoga we expand the possibilities for healing and transformation for ourselves, our communities, and our world.

Interlude: Building the Toolbox

This book aims to inspire a lot of thinking; interspersed with these big thoughts I drop little nuggets of *movement* in the interludes. These interludes offer experiments that complement other forms of yoga—they are tools, ideas, applications, and invitations to further explorations of mind and body and spirit. In fact, much of what I include in *Demystifying American Yoga* would not be considered "yoga" at all. This book is about American yoga and creative/critical embodied practices and neither "America" nor the critical and creative can be contained by the boundaries of the U.S. or by the ancient practice of yoga—for better or worse. Maybe this book isn't about *yoga* at all. Maybe it is about *embodied movement*. Maybe it's about a distinctively American (r)evolution—messy, flawed, and irreverent at times, but ultimately necessary if America is going to face the future we have built. As Resmaa Menakem writes in *My Grandmother's Hands*, "We Americans have an opportunity—and an obligation—to recognize [and move through] the trauma embedded in our bodies…. This will enable us to mend our hearts and bodies—and to grow up" (294). Maybe this book is about a reckoning and a coming of age, a necessary set of changes, and yoga is just a means to spark this transformation.

*

Some of the practices in these interludes are well-known, shared widely, and taught in a variety of different ways; some are novel to my approach. Most everything is a jumping off point, an invitation, a new way of looking at what we do with our bodies and minds and how we do it. Everything in this book aims to give you tools to put in your toolbox, to inspire your own yoga and mind/body/spirit practices, to help you to find ways to move that move you.

As a fitness/dance/yoga instructor (and as a professor), I create new combinations and approaches almost every day. I encourage people to take my tools and add them to their toolbox. I don't own any movement, any yoga pose, any sequence, any choreography, any idea. No one does. No one can. What I create and deliver may have original moments, but it has all come from what I have learned and adapted from the many inspiring instructors, teachers, trainers, and educators whose classes and workshops I have taken over the past 25-plus years and from the many teachers, trainers, and educators who have inspired them. The chain stretches back to ancient times, and it is a long and variegated chain. While this is the reality of the practice of fitness/dance/yoga, it is not sanctioned by the American fitness/dance/yoga industry where the ownership of practices, movements, images, names, approaches, and brands has become more and more controlled over the past few decades. In my work—in this book and beyond—I seek to disrupt the way that business is done, to empower individuals, systems, and practices to grow and evolve. The American Yoga enterprise is stuck in the nexus of power-over systems of domination. Teachers and practitioners, visionaries and facilitators have to create the future of American yoga—we are all a part of this transformation.

I invite each of us to tap into our rebellious American spirit and to create what works best for our contexts and communities. We call yoga and other mind/body/spirit approaches *practices* for a variety of reasons. As you build your toolbox, I hope you will draw from a variety of sources, resources, ideas and movements—from this book and beyond. If something doesn't resonate with you, set it aside. Circle back. Spiral in; spiral out. You might find that as your mind/body/spirit evolves you become ready to explore new ideas and insights as well as practices that you never thought you'd be interested in or able to do. This is the beauty and power inherent in the kinds of things that people have done with their bodies since ancient times—to connect, to grow, to process trauma, to heal, and to survive. I use the shorthand term of *yoga* in reverence to the ancient roots of contemporary American yoga, but also because it is a term that has become familiar enough in American culture that people are, perhaps, more willing to try something called *yoga* than something called *embodied movement*. I use the term yoga as a jumping off point, and I use it to expand and explode—to reimagine and re-envision and demystify—what we think of as yoga. While American yoga is most focused on exercise and the body, yoga also allows us to access the *subtle body*: the ego, the mind, the senses, memory, the unconscious and subconscious, the energetic, and more. Yoga roots run deep, but what grows from them is a forest of possibilities.

Introduction

Yoga is serious. It is an ancient practice from South Asia/India and Africa (as well as "pre–Columbian cultures of the Americas," as Amy Weintraub notes [12]), though we are less likely to recognize its African roots. It is a deep philosophy, a spiritual path, an indigenous medicine. It is also a big business, a variety of brands, and an endless playlist. In the United States and around the world, yoga has been defined, explored, adapted, appropriated, exploited, and more. Yoga has served the agenda of the powerful while it is also used as self-care and spiritual balm for activists who fight many forms of oppression. And it has been transformed by people as much as people have been transformed by it. Yoga, like any other activity, has its fans, fanatics, and celebrities. It means different things, to different people, in different places. There's the vanilla versions and the deep, rich chocolate versions, the traditional and the trendy, the controversial and the revolutionary. Yoga can be an escape and a remedy. It can be internalized and it can be misunderstood. It can be glossed over or over-indulged. It can be a nose up in the air and feet dug deep into the earth.

Demystifying American Yoga aims to help the reader navigate the worlds of yoga with critical consciousness, but without taking ourselves, or the practice of yoga, too seriously. It aims to demystify and complicate and inspire. Its focus is on what yoga is in the U.S. and what it might be. It aims to give readers some things to think about as well as some practical and effective yoga things to do. This book recognizes that yoga is something, like anything else, to be used in moderation and in cooperation. And it assumes that yoga—in all its richness, contradiction, and evolution—is not just powerful medicine to heal individuals, but also powerful potential toward social and cultural transformation. Yoga as social justice is not a new idea, and the idea that yoga is more than a physical practice has been gaining traction in the American yoga community (and beyond). One of my goals here is to examine, explore, and ignite this potential.

When we talk about social justice in the U.S., there is always resistance and backlash. When we talk about social justice in relationship to yoga, there will inevitably be resistance, especially from those who prefer their yoga to be an escape. Some will read this book as blasphemy. Some will dismiss it as not true to "real" yoga. Some will say my appropriation is typical of American yoga (and it totally is) and of white women who teach yoga in America (and maybe it is). But I contend that there is no one true yoga and that yoga is not something that can be bottled, packaged, branded, owned, or sold—though plenty have tried. White people, most often rich white people, have taken many things that were not meant for them—from indigenous traditions and ancient arts to the very cultural practices created to survive oppression—and we have trivialized, romanticized, bastardized, and profited from these things. We have hurt people and killed people through our taking, using, and other power-over practices. Cultural appropriation should not be shrugged off lightly. As Americans—the recipients of the spoils of centuries of brutality, to say the least—we have to find a way to practice yoga without continuing to perpetuate these harmful systems. Consciousness is key. So is the body.

Our bodies are sites of contention but they are also sites of connection and understanding. This is especially true since the way we move our bodies, how we connect with ourselves and others, and how we heal ourselves, have no cultural boundaries and multiple, often overlapping origins. In fact, many of the most powerful mind/body practices have simultaneous roots in multiple cultures. White people have tapped them all through colonialism, racism, imperialism, and appropriation. Today, we have knowledge and practices because of these crimes. And the American fitness industry continues to package and repackage the ways we move our bodies as if these practices are new; it sells us solutions to the problems we have created. Indigenous individuals may have, at times, sold out their people and traditions to prosper or simply to survive. This is one of the stories of American yoga. We have long divided ourselves; maybe our mind/body practices are the very things that unite us. No one owns yoga—no one owns movement and breath or meditation and stillness—and these are at the heart of yoga's power. They are at the heart of our collective power.

If someone tells you that yoga is only one thing, only a finite thing with strictly drawn borders, that person has a narrow understanding that contradicts the very essence of what yoga has been and can be. More, they have probably turned you off of yoga forever. This unconventional book aims to turn you on to yoga—to mind/body/spirit practices, to embodiment and empowerment, and to spiritual exploration unfettered by religion—forever, wherever you are. This journey is not limited by time or space, by who you are or by the body you inhabit, or even by the type of yoga you do. Yoga, many have said, is for everybody, for every body, for every mind/body. Yoga is for individuals and communities. Yoga is for empowerment and transformation, relaxation and recreation. Yoga is multitudes. Yoga is.

That's the American (Studies) Way

My focus on *American* yoga stems from my experience—as a citizen and a scholar. I "do" American Studies; this is the way I make my living (as a professor) and it is my life's work. Critical interdisciplinary and transdisciplinary American studies, ethnic studies, cultural studies, and women's, gender, and sexuality studies have been my passion and my calling and this container continues to grow. I am a doctor of American Studies. Right about now you are probably super impressed. Or, maybe you are rolling your eyes—at least at the doctor part. Perhaps you are thinking that I've included this fact to impress my readers with my over-educated credentials, to gain some upper-handed position over my readers, to prove my supremacy on all subject matter that falls under the huge umbrella of "American." Not just the U.S.—we claim the term American in all its glory! Maybe you're assuming that my over-inflated ego will be the driving force behind my words. You might not be wrong. But I mention my credentials because they shape my perspectives and they are at the root of my love/hate relationship with my country of origin. I have spent a lot of my time reading, thinking, learning, teaching, conversing, and writing about "America" and my ideas about yoga are shaped by this experience. My yoga teaching and yoga-teacher training has co-existed with my academic teaching and Ph.D. training. They grew up together and there have been many times when I have had to hide or downplay my academic credentials in yoga spaces and many more times I have had to minimize my yoga and fitness work in academic spaces.

As I bring creative/critical tools to our understanding and practice of American yoga, know that this is a complicated, sometimes contradictory, process. I lay a foundation and circle back. This is a contested process. I do not enter this process flippantly. I do not take the weight of oppression and exploitation lightly. I do not deny my privilege or ignorance. Still, American exceptionalism is difficult to bypass. In *Liberated to the Bone*, Susan Raffo explains American exceptionalism:

> As old as the American Revolution, it's the story that there is something unique and unusual about the United States. The first free country, the most compassionate, the first full democracy, and on and on. The more generations your people have been here, the more likely this belief system, woven together with the perfectionist individualism of racial capitalism, is somewhere inside of you, guiding the levers of your thoughts [140].

It is difficult to untangle our own American exceptionalism from all of our ways of sensing, knowing, and being. Inevitably, my arguments about American yoga are guided by my levers, even as I critique perfectionism, attempt to connect the individual to the collective, and problematize the drive of racial capitalism.

The yoga we have shaped in the U.S. is contradictory, complicated, and convoluted. Much of American yoga matches our cultural models and assumptions, especially as it has morphed into social media spaces. In her book *Yoke: A Yoga of My Self-Acceptance*, Jessamyn Stanley argues that "teaching American yoga, especially in the age of social media, *is* a performance" (69). American yoga teachers are often performers first because they are providing a show that people are willing to pay for, just like we have been programmed to pay for our entertainment and any other exchange of goods or services. "They expect a show" (70). So many of us have to pay to play, to make a living. We live in capitalist America, so it's nearly impossible to escape this dynamic. But, as Stanley argues, "If you're doing it right, practicing yoga is where performance goes to die" (70). In part, this tension between practice and performance is one of the realities of American yoga because, in America, our value is defined by our appearance.

American yoga is a quick fix, a superficial celebration of "better bodies" and feats of superhuman strength and flexibility. It has been touted as the answer to all of our physical health problems (and increasingly our mental health problems as well) and as a salve to our spiritual crises. Yoga is a trend to buy into (literally and figuratively), an elite pursuit that intentionally and unintentionally leaves people out, a hotbed of corruption, and ripe ground for capitalist exploitation. We brand yoga and we use all sorts of capitalistic, imperialistic devices to grow our business or our community, or to gain followers, or to prop ourselves up. And, yet, yoga is so much more than this. It sustains and connects us. It heals us. It puts us in touch with our inner selves and our potential. It opens us to the experiences of others. Yoga holds contradictions that threaten to tear us apart at the individual and the structural level. This, too, is American yoga.

A Shifting American Paradigm

As I have been working on this book off and on over the past seven years or more, my yoga practice has transformed me. There has also been a shifting paradigm in American yoga (and beyond). More and more attention is being brought to the cultural appropriation of yoga, to predominantly white-bodied spaces, to exclusionary practices, and to social justice and accountability. Many campaigns, websites, social media posts, popular magazines, corporations, organizations, non-profits, books, and yoga teacher-training programs have been making the argument that yoga needs to be respectful of the roots and origins of yoga, that we need to make yoga more accessible to diverse American bodies, and that American yoga needs to be more inclusive of the people and cultures where yoga has originated and evolved. Agreed. But sometimes these conversations and initiatives create more division instead of connection, more resistance instead of progress, more shame and guilt instead of healing, especially in the realm of social media. In the spaces where we are most likely to find yoga—from popular media to our local gyms and studios—conversations about cultural appropriation and social justice are largely absent. Sometimes, like when I teach students about yoga and social justice, we are told that *politics* has no place in yoga. But politics is already there.

America has only become increasingly more divided between what we have constructed as a right and a left side of the political aisle. Ideologically, yoga is used by the right and the left for their agendas. On the right, yoga is appropriated as a technique to make more efficient killing machines out of our soldiers (and then to treat their PTSD) and to placate over-stressed and over-worked corporate employees. Many people on the right see yoga as propaganda for the left and cringe at the inclusion of "land acknowledgments" or the sharing of pronouns, both of which are becoming more common practices in yoga spaces. On the left, yoga has been used to sell ideologies that whitewash and distort cultural roots as well as to prop up the "good" white people who are "woke" enough to say the right things and to "call out" or "cancel" those who haven't caught up with the latest trends in wokeness. On the left, we attempt to preserve a purity of yoga that is just as socially constructed as anything else.

Neither side of the mainstream American political divide has managed to find the unity, love, or potential at the heart of yoga. Too often, conversations about American yoga are limited by the dominant paradigm of privilege and assumptions that map along lines of racial groups, transferred onto individual bodies. These maps, which increasingly define contested American cultural spaces, reinforce dichotomies of white and black or white and BIPOC—almost always posing white as problematic and non-white as automatically "woke." Race is not so simple. As Susan Raffo explains, "Being raced means having the complexity of your history, your culture, and your understanding of yourself and your kin aligned with a category you have no power to shift. The only people who get to move into adulthood and experience life without the awareness of being raced are white people, even as white people are as raced as everyone else" (36). Here, in the U.S., we're all breathing the same air—the smog of cultural racism and white supremacy. As Beverly Daniel Tatum explains, "the cultural images and messages that affirm the assumed superiority of whiteness and the assumed inferiority of people of color—is like smog in the air. Sometimes it is so thick that it is visible, other times it is less apparent, but always, day in and day out, we are breathing it in" (65). Because we are all breathing the same air, we are all impacted. Tatum wrote this brilliant analogy long before the era of Covid (in 1997). The pandemic brought attention to the ways in which social inequalities exacerbate the problems of the air we all breathe. When we notice that there is a problem with the air, we can begin to mask ourselves to its effects. But we don't all have the same access to the tools that we need, which is why we need to work together. Together, we can begin to filter the air and address the root causes of the smog. Yoga provides a variety of ways in which our breath can be a tool but social inequalities limit who has access to these tools as well.

Yoga gives us tools for holding space and sitting with contradiction. Yoga asks us to look within and to go beyond social/historical constructions. The shifting paradigm of yoga from just another form of exercise to something that provides medicine, growth, and social and cultural transformation for the mind/body/spirit—individually and collectively—is one that I had been waiting for. Early versions of this book sat on the shelf because I was too busy, but also because I lacked examples outside of my own experience. I knew I was not the only one whose yoga was a practice of consciousness-raising and transformation, but I struggled to make the connections between what I was practicing and teaching in academia and what I was practicing and teaching in my yoga and dance classes. Michelle Cassandra Johnson's book, *Skill in Action: Radicalizing Your Yoga Practice to Create a Just World*, gave me a glimpse, but in 2020 America had no choice but to wake up. When George Floyd was murdered—when his breath was stolen by the increasing pressure of a police officer's knee on his chest—white Americans could no longer ignore what had been happening right in front of their eyes for decades, for centuries. We're still reckoning with our consent and complacence.

The confluence of Covid and Black Lives Matter mandated change, however slowly this change creeps along. For instance, at my university, and within the larger University of Maine system, what is now called "Diversity, Equity, and Inclusion" was of little importance. Some of us did this work because it was our calling and it was part of our academic training, but there was little support or recognition of this work. After Floyd's murder, DEI committees were mandated and top-down initiatives were put into place. Scholarships were created in his name. Similar trends happened in American yoga. Jivana Heyman writes, "we saw a strong reaction in the yoga community. Many white yoga teachers started looking for ways to support Black Lives Matter. Some of it was effective…. But some of it felt performative and simply offensive" (140). Performative is too often the American way. We can do better. Yoga has tools to help us do better.

It is no coincidence that both the Covid pandemic and the impetus for the explosion of the Black Lives Matter social movement hinge on the importance of unimpeded breath. "I can't breathe" has become a rallying cry as well as a symbolic representation of injustice in the United States. Michelle Cassandra Johnson's book starts with the breath as well. She writes, "I came to yoga by way of the breath" (x). She continues:

> When someone has experienced trauma, the breath is the most useful resource to stabilize the nervous system. The breath sends a signal that all is well; everything is okay. In a culture that would rather my black body not exist, let alone breathe, this feeling of "all is well" has been more than illusive. From the moment that I took my first breath until now, I have been on a journey to find air, to create an expansive inhale and a deepening of experience with my exhale. This is how I found it:

Her story—her path to yoga—follows, and her book's preface concludes by reminding us that "no one can exist without taking action. Skill in Action" (xiii). Our breath is a connection to ourselves as well as others; it is a connection to transformation.

Breath is life and when we inhale, we create more space in our bodies and in our minds—and in our social and cultural institutions. When we exhale, we release what no longer serves us—in our individual and collective bodies. In the last few years, several groundbreaking books about yoga have been published toward raising awareness of racism, cultural appropriation, racialized trauma, and with the explicit goal of growing conscious action in yoga teachers, trainers, and spaces. For instance, Johnson's book has a 2017 copyright date, but the edition that I read was published in 2020 and it was expanded with new material and republished in 2021. Susanna Barkataki's 2020 *Embrace Yoga's Roots: Courageous Ways to Deepen Your Practice*, Gail Parker's 2020 *Restorative Yoga for Ethnic and Race-Based Stress and Trauma*, Jacoby Ballard's 2021 *A Queer Dharma: Yoga and Meditations for Liberation* (about Buddhism and yoga), and Jivana Heyman's 2021 *Yoga Revolution: Building a Practice of Courage and Compassion*, all provide a wealth of insight into the shifting American yoga paradigm. I value the experience and wisdom of these yoga teachers/authors and each book offers a kind of self-study and deeper education about yoga. Each considers the ways in which yoga can address the ills of modern society and contribute to movements toward social justice. To do this work yoga must continue to grow and evolve while also providing space and opportunities for embodied movement for every body.

Through my teaching, and through *Demystifying American Yoga*, I attempt to humbly enter the conversation, which is moving too fast for any one book to keep up with. In the spirit of diversity and authenticity, the ways in which I practice and teach and write are all a product of my own unique American experiences and insights—the privileged positions I sometimes occupy and the aspects of my identity and politics that keep me from full acceptance, the trauma I have survived, and the critical interdisciplinary education that has shaped my life and worldviews. We all have unique and ordinary experiences. We all have more to learn. No one is born "woke," regardless of the color of their skin. Feminists are made, not born, as bell hooks' famous saying quips. There are no easy answers or simple ways to be conscious, alive, connected, authentic, and empathetic. But yoga does offer us one multi-pronged path toward these qualities if we are willing to open ourselves to the possibilities. And, if we honor the fact that yoga means *union* and *interconnection*, then we begin to see that yoga is bigger than any container we might make to try to hold it.

*

If you're feeling a little lost or a little bit disgruntled, don't worry—we're just getting started. You should feel your feelings. It is impossible to approach any subject with neutrality. We can certainly make the effort to do so, and there are benefits to this approach, but even when we claim objectivity, we are ultimately human. We cannot help but be influenced by culturally constructed ideas that we are born and raised with. Our American socialization and enculturation happens across all of our institutions, especially through education, religion, and media consumption. Being aware of our biases is a much more fruitful approach, but even when we are aware of our own biases we have to remain critically vigilant and self-reflective, humble and empathetic. Land acknowledgments, pronouns, lists of identifiers, accommodation requests, acknowledgment of elders or teachers or sources are all part of yoga's left-leaning practice. But these are only *practices* in an imperfect system of trying to hear and be heard. The right may mock these practices, but they are practices that are meant to interrupt the assumptions that we make when we enter into community or conversation. The left could do better to practice these more consciously, as embodied rather than simply performed.

More About My Approach—Here and on the Mat

My bias is all over this book. I am a feminist, a cultural critic, a professor, a yoga teacher, an academic, a fitness instructor, a JourneyDance facilitator, and an American citizen. I am white-bodied, though my body has always been too big according to society's standards and expectations and I have suffered from disordered eating and body image issues. I am more or less middle class, though for well over a decade I have been the sole income earner in my household. Throughout college and graduate school, I bore the brunt of the stress of bills and taxes and budgeting and saving and not buying anything that might be deemed unnecessary. I am frugal as much as I am generous. I am a woman with cisgender privilege, but adrienne maree brown's description of herself as "a woman with some boy in me" resonates with me; I also "haven't found the language for that" (*Pleasure Activism* 5). Sometimes I feel like my masculine qualities are going to break out and take over, and I have begun to use she/they and she/they/we pronouns more publicly. In a search for the woman I take for granted, I have begun to explore ideas and practices that connect me to the feminine power of goddesses and witches. I am queer but with assumed heterosexual privilege since I have been married to a man for a long time and my introversion, upbringing, and trauma make it difficult for me to talk about sex and my sexuality. Throughout my life I have had the appearance and function of an able body and mind; like most Americans, I have also internalized ideas of ableism. The more I learn about disability, the more I work to unpack my own ableism and to support the ideas and work of the Disability Justice Movement. As I approach age 50, and as I become more embodied, I have also started to discover that I am not as able-bodied or as neurotypical as I have assumed myself to be. Perhaps few of us are.

Identity is complicated for all of us, yes? Awareness of other ways of being, of other language that can be used to describe ourselves, often opens portals for understanding our whole selves and the many parts of ourselves better. If there had been language and role models for different ways of being and understanding when I was growing up and coming of age, I would probably have understood myself differently. Over the past 30 years, gender and sexuality have come to be (re)understood as a spectrum rather than as a binary. Language to describe ourselves has expanded exponentially. However resistant some people are to these more expansive ideas, the language that we continue to cobble together only describes reality. Language is a lifeline.

I teach and preach the need for intersectional approaches to identity and problematize the tendency toward pitting groups and individuals against each other. When we make oppression a contest, we are playing right into the systems and structures of domination—what bell hooks has called white supremacist capitalist patriarchy and what others have called imperialism or settler colonialism or The American Way. I believe in our collective power to not only challenge, but also remake and reform these larger structures. I beat myself up too often about not doing enough in this struggle (and then sometimes I learn to forgive myself). Already you can see my academia-bred tendency toward big ideas and over-explanation despite my attempts to stay authentically rooted in practice and experience!

*

You might wonder what all of this has to do with yoga. You might also note that I am an over-thinker by nature. Perhaps you are too. (Perhaps we all are and the nature of our culture conditions some of us to think less, to think more narrowly, and to fear difference.) One of the magical powers of yoga is a calming of the "monkey mind." Moving meditation, a connection of the mind and the body, helps to slow the busy mind, to focus us so that when we think, we do so with more calm and clarity. But here I am giving away the biggest secrets in the introduction. There's a lot in this book, and I invite you to meet it where you are and to take it at your pace.

The lens I put on yoga is transdisciplinary and critical, playful and exploratory. I bring critical theories (like feminism) and humanities approaches (like metaphors) into yoga practices, and I like to push yoga outside of its box. I have strong opinions based upon many experiences—on and off the mat, in and out of the classroom, and in and out of the fitness and yoga studio. I do not think that my perspectives are the only perspectives on these topics—not even close—and many of the ideas in this book will rub some readers the wrong way. People with similar experiences or disparate experiences will most likely agree and disagree with my arguments. Some readers will bristle and wiggle, deny and ignore. This is part of the uncomfortable, and even painful, experience of learning. We all have to make our own paths and make up our own minds, but our path and our mind both need some plasticity and some community. And this is exactly one of the points of this book. I challenge, interrupt, crack open, tease, expose, interrogate, and I ask my reader to do the same. This book is a conversation that unfolds through your reading and thinking as much as through your conversations and embodied experiences outside of this book.

Ultimately, the insights in this creative/critical yoga book are what you make of them. Progressing through each part—Discover and Practice, Unpack, Imagine, and Play—and in each Interlude between sections, there is space for exploration of ideas and space for contemplation, reflection, and meditation. There are suggestions for movement and prompts for beginnings. There is the opportunity to consider, or reconsider, physical poses (*asanas*) and mind/body/spirit practices. There is the invitation to shed new light on mindfulness and embodiment and what exactly this thing is that we call yoga. Each part adds layers, contexts, and tangents. Throughout, there are resources to continue your self-study beyond *Demystifying American Yoga*. (Self-study is also a practice of yoga, but we'll get to that later.) What you find in this book might surprise you. What you find in this book might challenge you. What we find in this book may surprise us. What we find in this book might transform us.

Interlude: Just Breathe

Because breathing is such a basic building block of yoga, we need some more information about breathing before we embark on this journey through creative/critical insights. In fact, I suggest that you keep coming back to this interlude—coming back to your breath—as you read. If you find your mind getting a bit agitated, just breathe. If you find uncomfortable ideas, just breathe. If you start to discover aspects of yoga you never imagined, just keep on breathing.

Even though I know about the power of the breath—through practice and study—I sometimes take its magical powers for granted. I get absorbed in a task—usually sitting, or slumping to be more accurate, at the computer—and then I will read my students' posts where they echo back my teachings, and I will sit up straighter and fill my lungs. When I got Covid, at the start of the 2023 fall semester, I found that my relationship to my breath changed like never before. I could not take a full breath. At the end of the same semester, my xiphoid process and rib slipped out of place, causing excruciating pain. My diaphragm was caught in spasms. Again, I could not take a full breath. And then I got the flu as the next semester started (it was a rough stretch there!) and, again, I had trouble breathing, which was compounded by a wicked cough that also kept me from sleeping. I was entirely dysregulated from stress and pushing myself, pretending my body did not exist. It is easy to get stressed or anxious and to forget to breathe. Our bodies breathe for us, so we don't have to think about it. But like all things in life, the more conscious we are, the more we get out of our experience. This is especially true for breathing.

The Power of Breath

Yoga, in its simplest form, is conscious breathing. Bringing attention to breath is yoga that anyone can do, and it reminds us of this basic building block of life. When we make the link between the mind and body through our breath, we have already transformed our breath. We have accessed the power of awareness and the tool of breath.

Too few Americans pay any attention to their breathing—unless something goes wrong with that breathing or unless they practice yoga. Some of us are afraid of yoga and we are afraid to breathe because when we breathe, we have to slow down. When we breathe, we have to listen to our bodies. We have to be present and embodied. For many of us, it seems much easier to just keep pushing through pain and discomfort and to keep breathing shallow breaths that only exacerbate our anxiety and disconnect. For instance, several students in my academic classes reported that they did not enjoy an activity that I asked them to participate in and reflect upon because, they said, it was too much like yoga. They had asthma and the moment they were asked to pay attention to their breath, they panicked and resisted. They had already formed a bias against yoga because of their past experiences. Even when I was not asking them to do yoga, their relationship to their breath shaped their experience coming into a practice that simply asked them to pay attention. When I told another group of students about this feedback from past students, a few who have asthma said that their experience was quite the contrary. Yoga breathing helps them to breathe better and to control their asthma instead of letting their asthma control them. When we take the reins of this autopilot tool, we might just find more power and empowerment—in our breath and in our lives!

Breathing is simple, but it gets so much more complicated. Many books about breathing are available, from the mystic to the scientific. I offer some basic breathing activities, but there is so much more. Sometimes breathing instruction is just "in through the nose out through the nose," but sometimes the breathing instructions given by an instructor suggest a breath that is too fast or too complicated to keep up with. If an instructor does not mention breathing, then you are really just stretching and not doing yoga at all. I most often instruct participants to inhale and exhale, matching our breath and movements or encourage them to just to breathe and move. Powerful breath does not need to be complicated. An understanding of breath and breathing is developed through practice—noticing, imagining, embracing.

Conscious Breathing: Building Blocks for Transformation

If you are taking a yoga class that includes few cues or explanations to guide your breathing, you are getting only the most superficial benefits of yoga. Yoga—at its best—is about a coordination of breath and movement, and at its core is the practice of conscious breathing. In other words, we want to pay attention to our breath and use it to support our movements, however big or small. A focus on the breath is a conscious breath and when we pay attention to our breathing we are already changing it. When we pay attention we can remember that the exhale is just as important as the inhale; we can also remember that breathing is a whole body process.

Just Breathe.
Just inhale and just exhale.
Tell yourself: Just (inhale) breathe (exhale).

*

Pay attention to your breath as you inhale and exhale. In through the nose, out through the nose. Let yourself take full, deep breaths. Just one will help, but try three in a row. If it feels good, try an exhale out through the mouth (like a big sigh).

Every breath is both the air moving in and the air moving out. The oxygen entering the body and the carbon dioxide leaving the body. (Pause and consider that plants are the opposite of our chemical exchange!) We often say breathe—meaning to inhale, but the exhale is key as well. The inhale expands our bodies and the possibilities in our lives, the exhale helps us to get rid of what we no longer need. Inhale in resilience; exhale out fear and doubt. Inhale in love for yourself; exhale out love for the people around you. Inhale in strength, power, and empowerment; exhale and find vulnerability and interconnectedness. Maybe you notice yourself relaxing with each exhale. Maybe there is clarity. Maybe only temporary reprieve. This is a start.

Our lungs are large organs and most of us do not take advantage of the full capacity and potential of our breath. We walk through our days keeping our breath constricted in the upper-most part of our lungs. This is a breath that contributes to anxiety. No wonder we are all so stressed out all of the time! Further, the less lung capacity we use, over time, the less we have to use. As we age, we lose lung capacity; when we practice yogic breathing techniques, we increase our capacity for life.

Now you have the tool. Any time you find yourself faced with unexpected stress or anxiety, pull this tool out of your yoga toolbox.

And build more awareness: notice where the inhale goes and try to let the breath naturally flow into the lower lungs. You might feel the rib cage expand into the sides of the body with the breath. You might notice the breath on the backside of the body.

Next: With each breath (in through the nose, out through the nose), try to lengthen the inhale and the exhale. Try to match the inhale to the exhale—the same amount of time for the inhale and the exhale. This is often referred to as equal ratio breathing.

Next: Try to lengthen the exhale. Let it last a bit longer than the inhale each time.

Next: Inhale through the nose. Then try pursing your lips to slow the exhale out, like breathing out through a straw. Research shows that a longer exhale reduces anxiety, but for me it often causes more anxiety. The more I practice the more I can embrace this tool of a longer exhale, especially if I imagine the straw or if I practice "bee's breath" where the exhale is a hum that vibrates the entire body.

When you're ready, you might pause your breath at the top of the inhale or the bottom of the exhale (called breath retention). Consider this a brief pause. Try one or the other—holding at the top or the bottom—and see what you learn through this pause. Like all things in life, it works better if you don't force it.

Make Some Noise

Just as some people are afraid to breathe, to let go, to listen to the body, some people are afraid to make noise. We hold ourselves so tightly. Natural body functions that make sounds are mortifying in quiet rooms and public spaces. With practice, breath is a means toward letting go. Letting go of stress, of tension in the body, of fear of the unknown. Letting go of past mistakes, moving through trauma responses. Breathe in, breathe out. Breathe in, breathe out. Breathe in, breathe out. What does your breath sound like? Maybe you notice the sound that travels in and out with the breath. If you plug your ears lightly, you might be able to hear your breath better; it might block out the world that is moving too fast, spinning around you.

One of the breathing techniques used in yoga is called *ujjayi* breath and is sometimes called "ocean breath," which helps make sense of how this breath should sound and feel. But we can also think about it as Darth Vader breath, which is perhaps not in line with the yoga principles and practices of *pranayama* (breath work), but is a fun cultural reference that will resonate with some (like me). One of my students wrote about how this breath reminds her of her favorite superhero, Batman, and how her brother once told her that she couldn't like Batman because she is a girl. Naming this breath practice as Batman breath was a fun way to help her feel seen and powerful.

This breath activates the parasympathetic nervous system, maintains heat, and slows the heart rate. It reduces anxiety. It also gives us something to focus on. Further, in the book *The Healing Power of the Breath*, Brown and Gerberg call this breath "resistance breathing" and describe how it is similar to a cat's purring, which makes it even cooler than Batman since I love cats way more than superheroes. When cats purr, it shows contentment. But more, purring *causes* contentment. The mechanics of *ujjayi* breath and purring are similar (33–4). Cats also purr when they are distressed and when they need to heal. A cat's purr is a healing frequency; it helps them heal and it can help us heal as well.

Ujjayi breath is relatively easy and simple. As you inhale and exhale, close the back of your throat a little bit. Imagine you are trying to fog a mirror. Pull the breath in with a slightly closed throat; release the breath gently and it "clouds" the ears.

My favorite noisy breath is bee's breath—inhale and then hum the exhale in any tone, or every tone. Feel the vibration in the body and maybe a tickle on the lips. Practiced in a group, this breath has powerful resonance.

Again, all breath work is best when it is not forced. And don't be afraid to make some noise.

Belly Breathing

One of the more challenging aspects of breathing—to understand and to practice—is what many call belly, diaphragmatic, or lower body breathing. This expansive breath makes space and relieves tension. It makes use of the full capacity of our lungs and the full range of motion of our ribcage. It expands the breath out and down into our diaphragm. I had to relearn this breath when I started seeing a physical therapist for pelvic floor dysfunction. I was breathing down into my belly, but I was bypassing my ribcage and not fully engaging my diaphragm. Thus, it was a shallow, incomplete breath. It was a disengaged breath. It exacerbated the tension in my pelvic floor. Like many breathing techniques, this one requires practice. It also requires us to let go, so don't try to force this breath. Let it grow.

We can start to further explore lower body breathing through yoga's three-part breath, which also takes patience and practice. Start with the hands gently resting on the chest, inhale and exhale. Notice the chest rise as you inhale; notice the chest fall as you exhale. Next, move your hands to the base of your ribcage. Feel the ribcage expand as you inhale and return to starting position as you exhale. Finally, bring your hands to your belly. Expand the breath down toward your hands. Notice the belly expand as you inhale and sink as you exhale. Then, put it all together, feeling each part expand with the inhale and relax with the exhale. Some of us teach three-part breath in the order of chest, ribcage, belly, as I have just described it. Others teach it as belly, ribcage, chest. Whichever order resonates with you is the best way to practice this breath. We might think about pulling the breath down into our belly like we are inflating a balloon, and then emptying the belly like we are deflating it. This kind of breathing takes some imagination.

Belly breathing is counter-intuitive to how most of us "naturally" breathe. Our paradoxical breath is not natural at all; it is a breathing technique conditioned by our culture. We tend to suck in our stomach with the inhale, a trick that many of us learn when we try to fit into that too-tight pair of jeans or when our mother or grandmother (or some other not-so-helpful friend or family member) tells us to suck in our unseemly gut. We suck in our guts all the time in an attempt to appear thinner, to fit in with the kind of body that society values, rather than the kind of body that is functional. Infants and singers already know the secret of the belly breath—the first unconsciously and the second through training and practice. The exhale can be a scream for attention or a beautiful melody—both are powerful!

Breathing the Elements

When I started practicing equal ratio breathing and other such techniques, I struggled with counting my breaths. I found that my counting would often speed up or slow down and had nothing to do with the length or the depth of my breath. I wondered if there were words that I could use instead since words resonate with me more than numbers and I realized that I have the perfect words for a 5-count breath: earth, water, fire, air, and ether/space. These are more than just words, they also inspire images and deeper resonance—they match with the elements associated with each of the chakras. So, as I imagine my breath, the five counts rise from the earth through the crown of my head, following the chakra path up the spine. Further, these words and images can be used to move the breath up the body: earth, water, fire, air, ether; and back down the body: ether, air, fire, water, earth.

I've also added movement to this breath sequence, which makes it more dynamic. Movement makes our bodies *and our minds* more dynamic. With this breath, we can feel our feet rooted to the earth on in inhale in mountain pose. With the exhale, we can bring our hands to our belly (water). We can float one arm out and down with an inhale and exhale (fire), and the other arm out and down with the next inhale and exhale (air). Then we can circle sweep our arms out and up with the next inhale, gathering the space around us (ether), and then exhale as we turn our palms to face our body, letting that all wash down the mountain and back to earth. Inhale in mountain, palms face forward, and the whole cycle of breathing with the elements starts again.

Whether numbers or words resonate with us, we can play with the ways in which we count and balance our breath. What words match your breath?

Heart-Centered Breathing

We can use our imaginations to visualize our breath, bringing love into our hearts and sending love and gratitude out from our hearts. We can grow love and compassion for ourselves and for others. We can place a hand on our heart center or layer the hands, one on top of the other, and feel the breath move in and out of our lungs. We can feel the expansiveness of our breath as well as the ebb and flow. We can lighten our touch with the inhale and gently press into the fascia covering the heart center with the exhale. Consider for a moment that the heart center includes the interconnected systems of respiration and circulation—the heart and the lungs. This nexus holds physiological importance as well as symbolic weight. "The heart is considered the source of emotions, desire, and wisdom" (Alshami). We put our hearts into the things that matter most. We wear our heart on our sleeve, signaling our transparent emotions. When we lose someone we love, our heart breaks. Scientific studies have revealed the connections between the heart and the brain, and the heart actually has its own brain or intrinsic cardiac nervous system (Alshami).

HeartMath provides a wealth of science related to the heart-brain connection. When we practice heart-centered breathing (or

HeartMath's "Quick Coherence" technique), we are, as their website argues, "Using the power of [the] heart to balance thoughts and emotions." And through this practice we "can achieve energy, mental clarity and feel better fast anywhere." We can feel the impacts of this breath technique without HeartMath's tools of measurement, but the science is an interesting bonus glimpse into concepts like heart-rate variability, coherence, and regulation of the nervous system.

*

All of the pranayama practices I share here are only the tip of the iceberg. There is so much more to discover and practice.

One

Discover and Practice

Each of us must discover yoga for ourselves, at the right time in our lives, in the right space, with the right people. But sometimes we might not realize that we are looking for yoga, let alone what type of yoga. We might not realize we are looking for something at all. We might be looking for love, self-acceptance, a way to burn calories, a connection in our community, a stress-reliever, a complement to our cardio or strength routine, a deeper meaning, or a new something to do. Or maybe we have found yoga and we are ready to go deeper. Yoga is wide enough to accommodate all kinds of searching. It is approachable enough to find a way in, and deep enough to keep us coming back.

My Discovery (and Ongoing Journey)

For a long time, I did not think I would like yoga. I knew very little about it. I thought about it as just a bunch of stretching. If I was going to work out, I was going to do cardio. Burn calories. I could stretch on my own if I wanted to. I was a fitness instructor, after all. I had all the tools. I learned the mind/body art of Pilates and thought its focus on the core to be superior to yoga. And then there was yoga's "woo-woo" reputation that turned me off. I am not a religious person and for a long time the most spiritual I would get was admiring the rugged beauty of the outdoors. But, after taking my first training—level one of YogaFit's teacher training program at a studio in Spokane, Washington, in 2005—I knew I had discovered something special, even if I could not put words to this feeling. Even if I had not yet tapped the deep well of yoga. Even if I could not imagine what yoga had to offer.

It took me thirteen years to complete the 200-hour teacher-training toward Yoga Alliance's RYT-200 certification. Most yoga teachers take a 200-hour yoga teacher training in a much shorter amount of time; some do very little teaching during their training. Because I had a background in teaching fitness, after my training I almost immediately began teaching yoga classes. I taught more than 1,000 hours by the time I was officially certified. There were many times over my thirteen-year journey that I thought I was done with yoga trainings. I certainly never thought I would reach that 200-hour marker! I took trainings when they were available to me—when I had the time and money and access. Sometimes I had to travel hundreds of miles to get the trainings I needed. Reflecting back on this long journey to a weigh station of certification (jump on board for the next 300 hours!), I am glad that I had time to apply what I was learning, to let ideas marinate, to seek knowledge and experience from other sources—some from conferences and online programs and some from sources outside of the technical boundaries of yoga. Some of what I have learned about teaching yoga came from discovering deeper elements of myself. My diverse and extended experience has given me a variety of insights that make me an intuitive, creative, connected, thoughtful, dynamic and passionate yoga teacher. I teach from my body as well as from my training and experience.

All of my yoga experience happened while I continued to get my Ph.D. and to work as a professor while also teaching a variety of fitness classes like step, kickboxing, and cardio belly dancing. Yoga was another thing on the list, another skill. For a long time, I didn't have a "personal practice." I was busy, overcommitted, distracting myself from the elements of my life that distracted me from knowing and accepting myself. I needed yoga more than I knew, but I kept it in the realm of fitness. I was afraid to get too close because I was afraid if I saw my self too closely I would not like what I saw. Over the past five years or so I have been more committed to establishing, growing, and maintaining my personal practice if only because I can't not do yoga as a part of my ongoing self-care and self-study—and because it has also shaped my professional life.

For years I kept my fitness world separate from my work in academia. In my 2014 book, *Women and Fitness in American Culture*, I wrote about my work in fitness and documented the merger of these two worlds. Much of my fitness story—at least the yoga part of this story—is re-told and extended in *Demystifying American Yoga*, but through a new lens and with unforeseen developments in my evolution as a scholar/activist, yoga teacher, and a fitness/dance instructor. After finishing a relatively complete draft of this book, my relationship to yoga expanded when I took module one and two of Journey-Dance teacher training in 2022 and started looking at the "spiritual" aspect of yoga (and life and dance and embodied movement) in new ways. (I dramatically revised and rewrote a new version of *Demystifying American Yoga*!) Several months later, I found myself opening The Spiral Goddess Collective, a Center for Mind/Body Movement, becoming a business owner and, as my mother insists on reminding me, an entrepreneur. I am not just a teacher anymore. I curate space for other teachers. I hold (and finance) space for community.

Ultimately, the most fundamental part of my personal yoga practice is teaching. Being a student is the best thing about being a teacher and being a student is a necessary way of life—in and out of yoga. I mix and match, build and create, adapt and adopt for my own mind and body as well as with the intention of sharing what I learn and encouraging participants in my classes to learn and grow as well. In this work, my yoga is activism—nascent and exploratory and seeking transformation of individuals as well as communities and (if I can be an arrogant American) maybe even the world. Yoga is my community service; it is my way of life. And yoga is a gift that keeps on giving and giving back.

Your Discovery

Your discovery may already be in progress. It may seem old and tired. It may be only in theory, or only in the first few pages of this book. It may be a few sporadic videos or the class you took that turned you off. You might have already realized the personal value that yoga holds for you, the positive impact of it in your life. You might struggle to make time for practice. Your discovery—of yourself, of yoga, of the world—is your life, your path, yours to shape and roll with. But we are all tethered to the same starting point, our felt, embodied experience. We can all come to yoga, and return to yoga, with eyes wide open.

All of the creative/critical insights in this book riff off of the many different books and writings about yoga that are readily available and growing with yoga's popularity, many of which lead to far greater range and depth about *yoga* than what I offer here. My *American* approach is part of the problem and part of the promise. I encourage you to read the books that I cite and highlight here and to search the internet for examples and topics, using my book to help cut through the bullshit and hype and navigate the complexity and contradictions. *Demystifying American Yoga* aims to give you points to pause, to maneuver, to explore; it does not aim to push or pull, only to move the reader forward—or sideways or upside down.

Excuses That Inhibit Discovery

There are a million excuses not to try yoga. I am sure I have heard them all. Perhaps the reader will recognize these familiar excuses....

- I am not flexible.
- I don't have time.
- I don't get a workout.
- I don't want to lower my metabolism.
- I don't have yoga pants.
- I am not religious or I am not spiritual (or I am differently spiritual).
- I tried it once and I didn't like it (which is not the same as I tried it once and had a bad experience with an instructor, studio, or one of the other people in class).
- I am not good at yoga.
- It moves too slow. I get bored.

- My body can't do the things that yoga requires (including being still).
- Yoga is too expensive.
- Only _____ people do yoga (fill in the blank: white, skinny, etc.).

All of these excuses are easily, but not flippantly, dismissed. Yoga does not ask anything of us except that we notice our breath and listen to our bodies. For some, this is a big ask.

Not flexible? Not only does it not matter, but since yoga grows flexibility, this is a particularly poor excuse. Don't have time? Since yoga can be done in many forms, variations, and durations, time is only an avoidance excuse. Yoga doesn't have to be an hour and a half class (though this is my preferred time span). Everyone has five minutes or one minute or at least the few seconds that a deep inhale and exhale takes. Yoga can be expensive, especially if we don't have access to free yoga classes or yoga videos (though many are available for free online … if we have access and know how to find what we're looking for). Yoga can certainly be intimidating for many reasons, and finding the yoga that is right for each of us might be time-consuming, frustrating, and exhausting.

Finding the right yoga can be a transcendent discovery. But yoga is not a religion. Some people might fear that the spiritual aspects of yoga run counter to their own religious beliefs, but spirituality is a wide open space—a container that holds all of those things that are bigger than us measly little human beings. Yoga may be spiritual to some people, but it is also a philosophy that complements all spiritual practices. Some people come to yoga searching for meaning and purpose. Some people find these things. Some people keep searching. Some people look too hard and miss the point and some people are knocked upside the head by epiphany or synchronicity when they are least expecting it. Thus, while some people come to yoga for the workout, they may be surprised or confused (or oblivious) when they find more.

The "workout" aspect of yoga is something that people chase or avoid or accept. Many kinds of yoga offer a pretty intense workout. While yoga need not be a physical practice at all, in the U.S. the physical practice is the most sought after—whether in pursuit of a "yoga butt" or "yoga body" or as a remedy for a day of sitting at a desk or chasing children or pounding the pavement—and the meditative, mindful aspects might be minimized or avoided in favor of the physical. The physical practice is how I first approached yoga; but yoga has changed my approach—to my workout, and to my life.

The one totally legitimate excuse not cited above, is the fear that comes from not feeling welcome in yoga spaces. While I would still argue that this excuse means that you haven't yet found the right yoga space, there are all kinds of reasons that we might not feel welcome in yoga studios. Sometimes those feelings are coming from our own insecurities, traumas, and fears. But too often these feelings are coming from unwelcoming spaces. Yoga spaces that are thin, white, cisgender, abled, and middle to upper class are often not welcoming spaces for people who do not fit into at least one of these privileged social classes. White spaces signal to people of color that this is not a space for them. Spaces full of thin women communicate that fat people are not welcome. Classes without modifications and options leave out all kinds of bodies (including my own). Fancy, pricey yoga clothing makes the person in sweatpants or Walmart-brand stretch pants feel like they do not belong. But, more than visual cues, these kinds of spaces also often come with attitudes and microaggressions that make the space unwelcome if not downright hostile. Gail Parker, Michelle Cassandra Johnson, and Susanna Barkataki share stories about how they have been treated in these kinds of yoga spaces. Well-meaning white people want to think that these kinds of experiences are exaggerated or that they don't happen as often as they do. Liberals and progressives often lament that "we are all one" or that *we* cannot force *them* to attend our classes. We might bend over backwards to prove how woke we are and how accessible our spaces are, or we might lash out at attempts to create safer, braver spaces for a particular group. We all have some more work to do toward social justice in yoga spaces—and beyond. Diverse and inclusive yoga spaces are harbingers of changing cultural norms that reach far wider than yoga studios. One thing that yoga teaches us (and Octavia Butler teaches us, as well as physics and myriad other sources): the only thing that we can count on in this life is that everything changes. Change is inevitable but we can shape change (says Lauren Olamina, Octavia Butler's protagonist in her *Parables* duology) and we can bend to meet the changes that might break us if we refuse to be flexible.

Mindsets That Inhibit Discovery

There are many mindsets that can inhibit the discovery of yoga. Some mindsets cause us to avoid yoga at all costs while others cause us to ignore parts of it and embrace other parts of it. Some mindsets cause us to skew yoga until it fits inside a comfortable box. One mindset that keeps people from yoga is the one that originally kept me from yoga. As a life-long fat girl turned fitness instructor, my focus was solely on cardio, cardio, and more cardio. Yoga meant wasting time that could be spent burning calories. This is a very common mindset, generally, and among fitness instructors as well. Or a version of it: it's just too slow. I need something more active. It's boring. This mindset makes me sad because I have seen many of my fellow fitness instructors and participants struggle with injuries that could be prevented or managed with a regular yoga practice. Or I see them try to burn away their anxiety or depression through hard core workouts. I want to give them the gift of yoga, but the gift of yoga can only be given to someone who is ready to receive it, even if they are not yet ready to embrace it.

While there is value in what Buddhists call the "beginner's mind," people who are new to something can struggle. Newbies haven't tried yoga, or have tried and have failed to find the yoga they were looking for. Newbies wonder what all the hype is, but they might be tentative to show up in a public space with other physical beings. Newbies panic when they hear *Sanskrit* or when they see a complicated pose. They are frustrated when they can't keep up with the flow, when they can't find their breath. They are frustrated when they are invited to feel something. These are all totally understandable responses. But the newbie who keeps an open mind will eventually find a comfortable fit.

There are some other American mindsets that prohibit the

discovery of yoga. These are not, of course, limited to Americans, but we are just really, really good at these mindsets: the cynic and the skeptic, for instance. The cynic has trouble relaxing with the idea of yoga, if not also the practice. The teacher's tone of voice, the glazed look in the eyes of the yogis, the seemingly blind adoption and adaptation of ancient cultures, the mindlessness that accompanies a pursuit of mindfulness. The cynic sees through the hype and wonders what else there might be to yoga beyond over-priced yoga pants and studios filled with skinny, snooty women.

The skeptic might want to believe in the power of yoga sometimes, but talk of energy and chakras (for instance) is met with a deep-seated doubt. When the teacher starts chanting, they are out the door—if not in body, then in mind. The skeptic may also fail to believe in the power of yoga to heal; they might doubt the scientific proof (which is pretty solidly established). Maybe the skeptic wants to be convinced, but resists.

Another American mindset that keeps us from yoga is perfectionism. So many people avoid yoga because they think: "But, I'm not *good* at yoga." Few of us like to engage in things we are not good at. Some of us—perhaps myself included—avoid those things like the plague. But yoga is not something to be "good" at; it is just something to be at. We have to let go of perfectionism, competition, and judgment—three key aspects of white supremacist American culture. We can't help but judge (ourselves or others), compete (with ourselves or others), or have unreasonable expectations (of ourselves or others). Expectations can negatively shape our perceptions and experiences. Our judgements can cloud our ability to see ourselves and each other in realistic terms. And our competitiveness can cause us to become injured and unable to practice, or unable to recognize cyclical progress, or even unable to recognize mental or emotional injury that accompanies the physical. (Note: letting go of competition, letting go of judgment, letting go of expectations is something that is taught throughout all of YogaFit's many trainings; it is part of YogaFit's "essence." These are mantras that have shaped my teaching and my life.)

Some people discover yoga and they just can't get enough of it. It becomes their drug of choice; they use it to fill the empty hole they can't otherwise fill. Addicts can't get enough of one thing, or many of these things: food, alcohol, drugs, sex, exercise, electronics, shopping, gambling, attention. They/(we) might flock to the promised therapeutic effects of yoga or may shun and avoid its tendency toward exposure of the deeper parts of the self. Addicts feed their soul through substances (or behaviors) that temporarily fill a void that remains just out of reach. Addicts can get that same high from yoga; yoga can be another abused substance.

Whether an excuse or a mindset, yoga can evoke fear. This fear may be more than just the usual fear of new or unfamiliar things. It might be a deep-seated fear, realized or not, that connects to past trauma. It may be an anxiety that arises from the idea of being vulnerable, in the middle of a group of strangers, in an unfamiliar and uncontrollable space and activity. It may be a fear of what we perceive as "religious" ideas that conflict with our own. It may be a fear of failure to perform or a fear of injury. It might be a fear of not fitting in, of feeling out of place. Of feeling like our body (or our mind, or our clothes, or our: you name it) does not mesh with our preconceived notions of yoga. We might feel like misfits. Misfits feel uncomfortable amongst a sea of thin, white, well-dressed people moving with a seriousness and purpose that makes them seem to be operating in a bubble. Misfits feel out of place in many places, for any number of reasons. Misfit is the wrong word. Or, it is the right word because it is our society's failure to accommodate difference and a spectrum of human experience that makes our culture—not the individual, not the body—the misfit.

None of these mindsets is an impossible barrier and some may be the best reason to discover yoga. I have been all of these and continue to manifest the cynic and skeptic despite my open mind and perpetual optimism. I have been a newbie to yoga, and continue to be like a newbie every time I try a new kind of yoga or a teacher or style outside of my comfort zone. I am a misfit—in body and mind—in mainstream American cultural spaces as well as traditional yoga spaces. And while I cannot consider myself an addict in the strictest sense of the term, sometimes that hole of disconnection and loneliness calls to be filled. And I have certainly struggled with disordered eating, codependency (or Robert Weiss's *prodependence*, as I prefer), substance abuse, negative thinking, and lack of boundaries. Many of us have at least a little bit of cynic, skeptic, newbie, misfit, and addict in us. And all of us need some new perspectives from time to time. Being in the right yoga space—physically and mentally—is key to overcoming limiting excuses and inhibitions. But finding the right space can be the biggest challenge to discovering yoga—unless we find that our body is the only space we need.

So What Exactly Is *Yoga?*

When we're talking about yoga, we're talking about a relatively simple thing and an extremely complicated thing. I might simply say that yoga is a combination of breath and mindful movement, performed through specific postures. But this is only one kind of yoga and is only scratching the surface. Most Americans know little about the eight limbs of yoga, connecting with the physical practice (*asana*) and maybe also with meditation (*dhyāna*) and breath work (*pranayama*). There is so much more.

In the first few lines of almost every yoga book, yoga is explained as "union." This is the literal meaning of the *Sanskrit* word *yoga*—to yoke—and can be as simple or as profound as a union of the mind and body or a union of breath and movement or the union of individual and community. In the first chapter of her book *Yoke*, Jessamyn Stanley writes about being called out by a reader for her "very specific typo" in her first book *Every Body Yoga*, defining the word yoga as "to yolk" instead of "yoke." She was mortified by this typo (been there!) and went on an emotional rollercoaster ride. This typo is enlightening if we consider that an egg's yolk contains protein-rich nutrients as well as the potential to create life. For Stanley, the situation led to part of what yoga is all about: "Yoga links the deepest and most conflicted aspects of [ourselves]. The light and the dark. The bad and the good. The ups and the downs. It's both a process and a destination, both a question and an answer" (8). Because American culture encourages us to think in binaries, yoga is a powerful tool to help us to think, move, and live with more depth and complexity. Maybe it can also help us let go of the little things—like typos!

Yoga is both an ancient philosophy and a modern therapy, a physical practice and a spiritual experience. What yoga is—where, when, to whom—is a matter of context and perspective. Yoga has been many things to many different individuals and groups. It has evolved over thousands of years and the physical practice has quickly evolved in the United States. At times in the history of yoga, the physical practice was seen as preparation for meditation and meditation was the primary practice of yoga for many people. At times— for a long time!—yoga was only practiced by men and boys. At times it was used as a kind of sideshow magic performance. Yoga was a means of resistance by Indians to British colonization and yoga was also a tool used by British colonizers. And when it came to America, yoga was first and foremost taught to the rich and influential—those who could afford to pay for promises of enlightenment and physical perfection. These American roots persist.

When we try to pin it down, yoga becomes more slippery. When we try to own it, yoga becomes too big to hold. When we try to preach instead of practice, yoga becomes empty and contradictory. Yoga is many different things simultaneously. No one yoga is more real or more right than the other. Plenty of people will defend the "real yoga" as thousands of years old, rooted in ancient (or contemporary) India. However, this yoga was one beginning, and if we romanticize and idealize some kind of untainted ancient yoga as the only true form of yoga it can take a form of something that never really existed or become inaccessible and exclusionary. Wherever and however yoga began in ancient India, it has continued to change and evolve—in India and beyond. It will continue to change and evolve within and without borders. Yoga's universality is part of its appeal and lasting power.

One example of yoga's evolution—globally and in the U.S.— is the story of Susanna Barkataki, who was born in the U.K. to an Indian father and a British mother. In her book, *Embrace Yoga's Roots*, she claims an authenticity in her story of yoga, rooted in her family history and ethnic identity. In a 2020 blog post she defends attacks that she is "not Indian enough." Her "culturally mixed Indian and British heritage," she argues, does not detract from the fact that she is "not half of anything. I'm fully Indian." Barkataki's Indian identity is one reason why she "devote[s her] life so relentlessly to yoga as unity." She also writes that she is "an immigrant to the U.S. because of violence targeting my Indian brown body, culture and family" and that she faced more discrimination and violence after moving to the U.S. Like other non-white yoga teachers and practitioners, the cultural turn of 2020 gave her an American yoga platform and she has made a huge impact after not being "given any platform or placement in the Western yoga and mindfulness industry for the better part of two decades." In addition to the publication of her book, Barkataki created the Embrace Yoga online course and the Honor {Don't Appropriate} Yoga Summit. Barkataki is the Director of Education for Ignite Institute for Yogic Leadership and Social Change where she offers a 200 and 300-hour Embody Yoga's Roots Yoga Teacher Training program. She argues that Americans need to learn from South Asian and Indian yoga teachers, an argument that I will loop back to in the "Unpack" section.

*

We have very little knowledge of India in the U.S. beyond what we may have learned in school about Gandhi's non-violence and India's victory over British colonization. I remember watching the film starring Ben Kingsley in history class and being taught that Gandhi's tactic of non-violence influenced Martin Luther King, Jr.'s, non-violent tactics in the Civil Rights Movement, but we didn't learn much beyond those vague historical facts. Until I read Jacoby Ballard's book, *A Queer Dharma*, I had not really considered how India's history has impacted contemporary practices, teachings, and politics of yoga. Again, I can be a typical myopic, default American sometimes despite my efforts at critical thinking and conscious contextualization! Ballard delves into the historical and contemporary context of yoga's history at home in India, which is a good starting point for all of us ignorant Americans (see Ballard 140–3).

There are countless, diverse books that tell stories of yoga's roots and many American authors and teachers make ancient ideas more accessible. In her foundational book *Living Your Yoga: Finding the Spiritual in Everyday Life*, Judith Lasater shares life lessons through yoga wisdom in the context of navigating modern life as a white, middle-class woman. She provides insights regarding discipline, letting go, self-judgment, faith, compassion, fear, patience, suffering, connection, service, nonviolence, and love. Each chapter centers on one of these and she provides practices and related mantras to help the reader navigate. Many of the lessons she shares come from the things that her children have taught her. She explains, "I like to say that I have several gurus, and they share my last name!" (99). Lasater's approach to yoga certainly resonates with mainstream America and she has been a shaping force through her books, trainings, and the reach of *Yoga Journal*, which she helped launch in 1975.

For many yoga practitioners, the *Yoga Sutras*—a core text of yoga philosophy and collection of oral wisdom that was compiled and written down by Patanjali sometime in the ancient past, between 500 and 200 BCE, if you ask Wikipedia—are a key to understanding what yoga is. Another version of this story cites the origins of the *sutras* as the notes that Patanjali's students took as he shared his wisdom orally. Some have postulated that Patanjali was not a single person, but several people with the same title. Many translations and interpretations of the 196 *Yoga Sutras* exist and they are considered to be the foundational ideas of the ancient science of yoga. They are meant to be studied, meditated on, memorized, and revisited over the course of a lifetime. The *Sutras* ("threads") have plenty to offer anyone and everyone in our modern world, even (or especially) shallow Americans like me. For me, the *Sutras* are mostly esoteric, dry and boring. They remind me of reading the Bible or Shakespeare—classic texts I do just about everything I can to avoid (sorry, not sorry). Regardless, the *Yoga Sutras* are an important aspect of the yoga tradition and are worth reflecting upon as a part of a life-long practice. I prefer interpretations to the originals. And there are plenty of interpretations to explore.

Jivana Heyman reflects on a variety of interpretations of yogic texts and philosophies in his book *Yoga Revolution*. He explicitly engages with a variety of translations and interpretations to get at the nuances of these ancient texts. He notes that "while the teachings are timeless and universal, our circumstances have changed. We have no choice but to interpret the teachings and apply them to this moment" (14). But, he argues, we also need to "be aware of our own prior conditioning and the way we have been trained to think and see the world" (14), which includes becoming "aware of our proximity to power and the ways we have experienced oppression, or not" (15). Both Heyman and Lasater seek to make ancient teachings relevant to our contemporary lives and landscapes, to make yoga accessible and more easily understood. (Heyman's first book is *Accessible Yoga: Poses and Practices for Every Body* and he is the founder and director of the Accessible Yoga Association, an international nonprofit and the co-founder of the Accessible Yoga Training School.) Both have devoted their lives to the study and teaching of yoga.

For a long time, my understanding of yoga was primarily experienced through my body and the yoga teacher trainings that I took through YogaFit. My further study is less mainstream and more academic, beginning with Carol Horton's book *Yoga Ph.D.: Integrating the Life of the Mind and the Wisdom of the Body*. Horton brings the practicality of the social scientist while trying to make sense of some things that just have to be experienced—to be felt through doing. Horton's book was one of the first books I read about yoga, after I read her co-edited book, with Roseanne Harvey, *21st Century Yoga: Culture, Politics, and Practice*, while I was researching and writing my book, *Women and Fitness in American Culture*. At that time, I had a lot more to learn about yoga. I still do. My self-study resonates with authors, teachers, and practitioners who have shaped American yoga at the edges of the mainstream. I'm most interested in how America's teachers and practitioners have shaped yoga—for better or for worse. In her book *Yoke*, Jessamyn Stanley illuminates what she calls the *"yoga of every day life"* (15). This is American yoga. Most Americans practicing yoga are taking yoga classes, for any variety of reasons, but mostly because it make their everyday life better. Some go deeper, but going deeper requires effort and an impetus that is not often highlighted in American yoga spaces.

*

When we are talking about, learning about, thinking about yoga, there is no such thing as "just." Yoga is not just philosophy; it is not just stretching. And it is not just whatever one expert or another expert says it is, no matter how authentic the source may claim to be.

In order to understand American yoga as multidimensional we must see beyond misleading American myths and superficial practices—in and beyond the glossy, digitized world that dominates American yoga consciousness. *Demystifying American Yoga* explores the possibilities of what yoga means, universally and personally. It comes to no specific conclusion about the nature of the beast except that yoga is a practice so vast that it can contain its own contradictions. At the same time, I argue that yoga is scientifically sound as well as eternally ethereal. Yoga is also a practice so personal that we need to understand some of the nuances in order to get the most out of our practice. But collectively, and in community, there is an under-tapped power. Instead of—or in addition to—asking what yoga is, we might be better served by asking why we need to *practice* yoga.

Why Do We Need to Practice *Yoga?*

There are many answers to this question, and some of these answers really can't be put into words—why we need yoga must be felt, experienced, and embodied. But the short answer: to become more flexible and better balanced, to slow our minds down and to listen to our bodies, to connect our minds and bodies, to move and breathe in ways that calm our nervous system. Yoga can be a totally relaxing and rejuvenating experience. It can also be hard work, full of push-ups, squats, and plenty of sweat. I prefer the former but America's fortune is founded on the latter. Even those practitioners who embrace yogic philosophy and spirituality sometimes have trouble letting go of the very American "no pain, no gain" approach to yoga, as Judith Lasater describes in *Living Your Yoga*: "Throughout the years I have noticed the tendency in myself and others to think that we must practice boot-camp yoga—that is, the poses must be difficult even painful, to be beneficial and worthwhile" (33). The lesson here is that "our thoughts about the poses reflect our thoughts about ourselves" (33) and this example of self-judgment is toxic to our bodies and minds and to our lives and the ways that we act and interact in the world. Through yoga we can learn to find comfort in yoga poses instead of pain and while "the difficulty [of yoga and of life] might never change ... your attitude and inner dialog can" (37). There is no mindset as judgmental as the American mindset and many of us are so used to beating ourselves up and cutting other people down that we don't even realize that there might be another way. Yoga reminds us that we can change our minds at any time. Literally.

The longer answer to why we need to practice yoga is part of the explanation offered by the whole of *Demystifying American Yoga*, but it is really so much bigger than any one answer or any one book can contain. Yoga has physical and mental benefits, and even when we choose yoga for one particular reason, even when we focus yoga on this goal, the other benefits are going to creep into the equation. For instance, the athlete who does yoga might want the physical challenge, a complement to other fitness goals and skill sets, but the mental strength and emotional release might be just as beneficial for athletic performance and yoga might also help injury prevention and healing.

Yoga can foster physical flexibility, but perhaps mental flexibility is a more profound effect. People who are naturally flexible might be able to contort their bodies in ways that amaze and astound the less-flexible masses, but if yoga is not done mindfully, a hyper-flexible individual can injure themselves. If we focus on the physical, we may overlook the deeper introspection that comes with sitting with oneself in tension. The woman in a yoga class who can touch the floor in triangle pose might get more out of the pose if she chooses not to touch the floor. The man who always chooses the full side plank might benefit from the different balance challenge and stretch of modified side plank. The person who rolls up their mat and tiptoes out during final relaxation might be missing out on an already too-short moment of stillness and breath. Yoga fosters mental flexibility so that we are willing to try new shapes as well as new ways of seeing and being, of loving and living.

There are many more possible answers to the question of why we need to practice yoga. Some of these answers are personal and some are for the benefit of the collective (or both!). In an "Integrative Healing Yoga" class that I teach for nursing students, the why takes on a variety of dimensions from self-care to a holistic "whole person" approach to health and wellness. The wealth of scientific, evidence-based research gives them the proof they need to satisfy the Western skepticism of "alternative" medicine. Yoga is a documented tool for treating or managing low back pain, ADHD, type two diabetes, high blood pressure, depression, anxiety, PTSD, and more. But in addition to the students' research, they also experience the benefits of yoga through practice—as a remedy for the physical and emotional toll of doing the work of nursing. Most students enter this class with little to no yoga experience. Many think yoga is about skinny, fit women in expensive clothes who bend themselves into pretzels. By the end of class they have an arsenal of tools. They spread the message—the answers to the question of why.

Getting to Know Your Body

One answer to the why of yoga is access to body awareness. In America we are obsessed with the way we look. We pride ourselves on our appearance. We judge our performers and our presidents based upon the way that they look. We keep ourselves from doing the things we want to do because we are afraid we might be judged by the way we look. We are not wrong. American culture is a cold, judgmental, narrow place most of the time. Getting to know our bodies requires going deeper than surface appearances. I find that many of my yoga participants appreciate the lack of mirrors in a space where we are practicing yoga. But other students lament the lack of mirrors because they want to *see* if they are doing the pose correctly. *Seeing* their body is (they think) the best way of *knowing*. While there is value to being able to see ourselves doing a yoga pose, and to make adjustments based upon what we see, what we *feel* in a yoga pose is far more important. Since we aren't often taught how to feel our bodies in space, this is a tool we have to develop. And yoga can help to teach us this body awareness from the inside out and the outside in.

In the U.S., and in the West more generally, we have looked to (medical) science for an insider's understanding of our bodies. Raffo exposes the hidden story behind the body knowledge contained in books and online resources: "This thing we call anatomy, this wealth of information catalogued on the page, this compilation of drawings, recordings, and objects floating in formaldehyde, evolved out of a mix of slow observation and violent attack" (39). Even our basic understanding of our bodies and their systems and structures are a part of our violent history. Thus, Raffo argues, "How we talk about—and experience, connect with, care about, live in, and attend to—bodies matters" (39). Too often our understanding of our bodies is superficial, incomplete, and skewed by the messages and misleading information that we are bombarded with. We don't need a college-level education to understand some helpful basics. Paying attention is a good start. As Raffo argues, because of the violent origins of our basic knowledge, "It's important to the path of liberation and to honoring the sovereignty of individual bodies to have their own experience of themselves" (39). Embodied practices like yoga can help us to develop our own experience of our bodies as they move through space and provide us with the only home that we can ever freely inhabit.

There are also coloring books and online resources that provide different ways of learning about the body. Ann Swanson's *Science of Yoga: Understand the Anatomy and Physiology to Perfect Your Practice*, is packed with information and full-color illustrations of what the body is doing in each pose. When we know the basics of the body we are better prepared to move, meaningfully and consciously. The basics of the body remind us that we are flesh and blood, muscle and fascia, bones and sinew. We all have these basic building blocks in common. However, as Susan Raffo explains, "anatomy is a map that helps give you a sense of the general layout, but when you go looking, things are often not where you thought they would be" (39). Our bodies are unique on, as well as below, the surface of our skin. They are shaped by our experience, our history, and our relationship to our own bodies. This is one reason why she advocates for thinking about "anatomy as poetry rather than as steady fact" (39). (I'll come back to this idea later.)

Exploring Practice and Self-Study

There are many ways we can think about the *practice* of yoga. Perhaps most obviously, we might call it practice because there is no need for competition, no necessary end goal. It is process—the mental and physical prep for the game, not the game itself. Of course, many people make yoga into a competition—and not just Americans. Whether it is the competition we find in our heads as we look over at our neighbor's yoga mat, or the international competitions where poses are scored and winners are named, competitive yoga exists despite what the *Sutras* may teach and the yogis may preach. When we compete within the world of yoga, we may lose some of the essence of yoga. Yoga is a way of being, a way of thinking, a way of living. It can only be practiced, not attained. It is learned in layers and sustained over a lifetime, even if practiced sporadically. And, again, because conscious breathing is the simplest form of yoga, any time we are paying attention to our breathing, we are technically practicing yoga. In everything, we can only *practice* because no piece of art—no person—is ever complete. The old adage of "practice makes perfect" is, perhaps, overstated. Practice doesn't make us perfect, but maybe it gets us as close as we can get. Ultimately, practice is process. We don't need to bend our bodies into unfamiliar shapes without being invited into those shapes by our body and our mind.

I like to think about the practice of yoga as a practice of sampling: something new created with a familiar loop. We recognize; we riff. We remix. To do this, we have to borrow from the source, but then we make something new. In the best sampling practices, we honor the original source, but sometimes that source wants recognition or compensation. In everything there is negotiation, a give and take. Educating ourselves about the different styles, approaches, and philosophies of yoga is a first step toward creating our ideal—and flexible, evolving—mix. Sometimes the list of yoga choices seems impossible to navigate. To make things more confusing, the same words may be used to describe vastly different styles. And yoga brands attempt to own and contain yoga—to limit the yoga experience to the brand, to the promise to "shred" or "burn," for instance. And to top it off, different teachers may teach the same style and still teach drastically different classes. I have witnessed many people search for yoga and find themselves in the wrong space and place. Sometimes they try again. We should always try again. Even if we already do yoga, we can practice the beginner's mind concept. When we approach something as beginners, with an open mind, we learn new things or we re-learn things, or we learn things in new ways. We shore up our foundations and continue to build. Most importantly, if it feels good, do it. If it doesn't feel good, don't do it. Lessons for yoga, lessons for life.

I find constant sources of new inspirations and new possibilities and that is part of what I love about yoga. Self-study is called *svādhyāya*, one of the *niyamas* of the yoga philosophy. *Demystifying American Yoga* is an exercise in *svādhyāya*. It is one of many road maps on each individual's yoga journey. It encourages us to explore: books, videos, blogs, websites, classes, workshops, events—all sources that help us grow. We might focus on history, philosophy, medicine, the subtle body, and learning about the Eight Limbs. But while self-study is shaped by the needs and desires of the individual, it is also shaped by the world that we live in and the realities that shape all kinds of experiences with—and beyond—yoga. Most self-study requires going within rather than focusing on what is going on outside of ourselves. Again, if the rich Eastern philosophies are what float your yoga boat, there are many places to dive into the depths. This is America, baby. I'm only trying to skim the surface and give you something to chew on. This feat alone is vast. Self-study also means looking at the bigger picture, looking deeper and further than our individual selves and our limited sight, our culture and our limited ideologies. Self-study means that we can't just do yoga. We also have to think about yoga.

Why Do We Need to Think About Yoga?

Skimming through life in a blissed out state is not what yoga calls for. Yoga is deep and wide, ancient and contemporary, diverse and evolving. If we don't think about what we practice, if we don't choose to go deeper, then are we even really doing yoga at all? Privilege—not yoga—allows us to tune out the voices, ideas, people, and challenges we don't like or we don't want to deal with. At a yoga training I attended years ago, one of the women said that she had chosen not to watch the news (and this is before the news got really, really hard to watch!). I understand. I understand the need to distance ourselves, at least temporarily, from things that drain our sanity and threaten our mental health. And the news, in its sensationalism and selectivity, is toxic. Overindulgence in the news that spews from white supremacist capitalistic-driven 24-hours news cycles certainly fucks with our heads and our hearts. But choosing to detach, to tune out reality, is a privilege that too few can afford. Reinforcing our own limited version of the world is something that Americans are really good at doing—on the right and on the left. Perhaps I am as guilty of this as anyone else.

Our privilege to tune out the news is in stark contrast to the people whose lives are broken and exposed on news programs, only to be ignored by those of us who can afford to look away. This kind of disengagement—the privilege to look away, to close our ears and eyes—is only a temporary fix; it only makes us feel better as long as we can keep the negative at bay. But the negative is a natural part of life. Bad things exist. Bad things disproportionately impact the most vulnerable people in our world. When we ignore our privilege, we ignore other people's oppression. Our privilege only exists because oppression exists. Our ignorance perpetuates and even exacerbates the negative things that we think we can afford to ignore. We should not feel guilty about this fact; we should feel responsible to help change it. Yoga's "positivity" or "positive thinking" can't ignore, but it can remedy. And it takes more than meditation and donations to make a real-world impact.

The world is a complex place full of pain, corruption, and greed. This is a lot to think about and yoga can help us think about our world with more empathy and compassion. We don't have to solve these problems through yoga—in fact, we *cannot* solve these problems through yoga. The world is also full of love, acceptance, and compassion. Yoga can help us tap into these positive aspects of our world. If we choose to use yoga as a means for escaping the truths of the world we live in, if we use yoga to escape to our comfortable corners, if we refuse to acknowledge the ways in which we are implicated in the misery of others, we are not only doing a disservice to our world, we are also doing a disservice to ourselves. Thinking about yoga—and thinking about yoga in new ways—is in the service of the spirit of yoga and our increasingly complex world. We might even think about service as an integral part of yoga. Some training programs, some instructors, and some studios include service in their mission. When we serve others, we make the world a better place and we make ourselves better people. But more on that later.

*

The ancient philosophies I touch upon in this chapter are only the very tip of the iceberg. If I am glossing over them here, I don't mean to demean or dismiss their importance; I am only admitting my lack of expertise in this realm of yoga. I am an Americanist, a futurist, and a bricoleur (someone who creates from a diverse range of sources). I come to my practices of yoga without apology. There is so much more. Every time we let a new idea settle and grow, another concept is there to extend the bridge to a better understanding of ourselves and our world. The Expand section is more than citation—it is an invitation to continue the yoga journey beyond this book. The layers, the resonance, the lasting influence, the new insights and interpretations—this is where the power lies. Study. Mix. Practice. Remix.

What I offer throughout the rest of this book are unconventional insights into American yoga. I ask the reader to journey with me as I unpack some of the myths and messages of American yoga—the good, the bad, and the ugly—and as I ask us to tap into our imaginations to discover the possibilities of yoga beyond the physical and beyond the ordinary and conventional. But before we dive head first into the rabbit hole, I provide an interlude with tools to further explore ourselves and to begin to embrace the "woo-woo" of yoga—the parts of yoga that many Americans are most skeptical of and maybe even a little bit afraid of. I certainly used to be far more skeptical than I am now, and I continue to evolve. Sometimes Americans are able to keep an open mind even while we remain a little bit skeptical and this is when we are at our best.

Interlude: Exploring Your Self and Embracing the "Woo-Woo"

This interlude provides tools for getting to know ourselves better, to explore ourselves from the inside out. Bo Forbes talks about how our body is our laboratory. We can also think of our body/mind/spirit as an endlessly fascinating puzzle. This puzzle, however, does not need to be solved; instead, we are just shifting and arranging the pieces to map a current understanding of who we are, where we come from, what we need, what we want, and what gifts we have to share with the world.

While this interlude includes "Embracing the Woo-Woo," in its title, I really don't consider most of this section to be "woo-woo" at all. There was certainly a time when I would have thought some of the ideas and practices here were way out in left field, and I would have avoided them at all costs. But what I have found through practicing yoga is that what seems impossible or improbable shifts when we learn to open our minds, look within, and let go of judgments and expectations. Life is full of possibilities and perspectives that we have collectively decided to jettison into the realm of "woo-woo." Here we are only taking the first steps toward broadening our perspective beyond the concrete, safe, and logical.

Upside Down Brings New Perspectives

While Americans have a well-earned global reputation as some of the most selfish and short-sighted human beings on earth—the most individualistic, arrogant, myopic, and self-centered—so many of us, especially women, people of color, queer people, and other marginalized folx, are hypercritical of ourselves. We lack self-confidence and have no idea how to love ourselves, even when we might project confidence or even arrogance. And who could blame us when we feel that our country and our culture do not have our best interests in mind, to say the least? But even the most securely positioned in our cultural hierarchies often lack self-confidence or, at the very least, lack a knowledge of self beyond what they are supposed to be. White men who deny the rights of immigrants, preach the glories of capitalism, beat the women they think they own, claim "involuntary" or "nonconsensual" celibacy (incels), shoot up schools, kill Black people who are out for a jog, and any host of other deplorable acts are, we might argue, at their core, miserably unable to live up to the hype of masculine, white supremacist patriarchal culture. They take this out on other people because they cannot face themselves or imagine a way of being and living differently.

If we all had equal access to the basic necessities of life—food, water, shelter, clothing, education, health care—and we were taught from an early age to listen to our bodies, to explore who we are and what interests us regardless of the gender identity assigned to us (or if we were not assigned a gender identity at all!), and to treat other people with empathy and respect, the world would be a very different place. If love, empathy, compassion, care, and justice were the driving ideologies of our culture, what kind of world would we live in? This vision would be considered idealistic and leftist to many Americans and we might expect to find such sentiments in a book about yoga! But there is nothing idealistic about this vision; it is a realistic vision—a real possibility if we want it to be. And many of us do want this vision. We just cannot agree on how to reach it. We have to stretch our minds to be able to see a world turned upside down. (The echoes of Lin-Manuel Miranda's masterpiece, *Hamilton*, are entirely coincidental here, but not irrelevant!)

One of my favorite cards (framed on my office wall, created by Leigh Standley of Curly Girl Designs) has an artistic image of a woman in wheel pose with the phrase: "Funny, she said, how sometimes right side up can come from upside down." While many poses (like down dog or standing straddle, for instance) include an inversion, there are specific inversion poses, most often done in the final section of class before final relaxation, like plow and shoulder stand. I avoid these two inversions because my breasts choke me. A simple inversion is all we need.

Any kind of inversion—when the head is below the heart—has health benefits (and cautions), but the simplest and perhaps most beneficial is the simple inversion of legs up the wall (or in the air). It's exactly what it sounds like. Sit down and scoot your side hip/booty up against the wall. Roll and bring your legs up like you are sitting on the wall. Use pillows or blankets underneath your lower back (or head) if needed for support or comfort or to lift the hips and get even more upside down perspective. Breathe.

We can add variations: open the legs to a straddle position, bring the heels together in a butterfly, add an upper body stretch.

If the legs up the wall is too intense of a hamstring stretch or uncomfortable, you can put your legs on top of the seat of a couch or chair (so they are at a 90 degree angle instead of straight). And, really, as long as your feet are higher than your heart, you're there. This pose is also great to lessen sciatica and low back pain, help balance blood pressure, aid with digestion, relieve tension and stress, improve circulation, relieve headache pain, improve sleep, help manage varicose veins, and increase energy.

The literal inversion of the head below the heart is what the physical yoga pose is about, but we might also think about what this means metaphorically. When we put our heart above our head, we commit to feeling more than thinking. When we look at things upside down, we have a new perspective on our surroundings, our culture, and maybe even on our life.

Personality Tests

In the quest to know ourselves better, a number of tools are at our disposal. These tools are lenses through which to consider ourselves and the world around us, but it is important to remember that these are all tools. One tool is psychology and, specifically, personality tests. For many years I thought that psychology was bullshit. Sociology appealed to me and made sense to me and that's what I focused on in college. Like the typical ignorant know-it-all, I skipped past intro to psychology and went into personality theory, but I did not take it seriously. Now I find psychology to be fascinating, and one of the tools in my toolbox, even though I still tend toward theories of social construction in most cases.

There are the most well-known personality tests like the Myers-Briggs Type Indicator (check out 16Personalities) and the Big Five Personality Test, as well as a variety of IQ tests and tests that are indicative of a person's strengths and abilities. Some of my colleagues are all about the Enneagram personality test, which systematically defines nine personality types (but gets way more complicated) and promises to reveal a person's core fears, motivations, and superpowers. There are also EQ tests that measure emotional intelligence. For fun, and character insights (pun intended), there are also a variety of tests that measure which Hogwarts house you belong to (via the *Harry Potter* Sorting Hat) or which faction you would belong to in the *Divergent* book/movie series. There are tons of these kinds of tests (and many are not necessarily informed by the rigors of social science). It can be easy to get lost in these quizzes (I just got lost in the Visual DNA test). Ultimately, all of these are simply tools that we can use to better understand ourselves while also recognizing that we are complex beings in a complex world and we are always changing and evolving.

The more woo-woo version of personality insights is astrology—charting time and place of birth and tracing the cosmic energies present when we emerge into this world. This is an ancient system with multiple origins that is practiced by all cultures and peoples in different ways. It is an art and a science. My practice and understanding is superficial and sporadic, but enlightening when I seek out a source or listen to a friend's knowledge of the Zodiac. Like most things, astrology gets way more complex; there are layers to explore beyond knowing what our sign is.

Astrology can be used as a tool and trend toward manipulation and as a means of spiritual bypassing or as an excuse for an unchangeable nature or bad behavior. But all tools have this application. Whether the results of a personality test or an astrological reading, nothing about us is concrete and unchangeable; we are malleable. This means we can be manipulated, but it also means that we can manipulate ourselves. We can change our shape. Thus, we should choose our tools wisely and apply them with a critical lens.

Meditation

Meditation is central to yoga practices where the physical poses are only bolsters for what the mind is doing. However, there are many different kinds of meditation and they are all different and all worth a try. We can't do meditation wrong, despite the feeling of failure many of us have when we can't clear our minds and drift in clouds. Our minds are busy and they often spin out of control as they anticipate the future, ruminate on the past, or try to remind us of all of the things we *should* be doing. This state of mind that so many of us share is exactly why we need to practice meditation.

Sometimes I envy and admire those who have a meditation practice that works for them. Sometimes I think successful meditators are just practiced liars. States of bliss can be imagined just as easily as they can be experienced. But whether the evidence is qualitative or quantitative, there are certainly physical and mental benefits to meditation—better sleep, reduced stress, better coping skills, managing anxiety and depression, developing concentration, and decreasing blood pressure, for instance. However, the way that meditation has been approached in almost every yoga class I have taken has been of little use to me. Sit on your mat. Sit comfortably. (Already, I fail. Sitting is rarely comfortable, especially if I have not moved and warmed up my body before sitting.) Straighten your spine. Focus on your breath. We're going to sit here and meditate for five minutes. And then we're on our own. And then we're told that the distractions of our bodies are only our minds trying to trick us. That pain in the shoulder. That itch on the shin. Distractions.

I didn't seriously try to practice meditation until I took a yoga training that focused on meditation and mindfulness. We were encouraged not to berate ourselves if we find our mind wandering.

Just bring the focus back to the breath. This was the first time that meditation felt accessible and the first time it resonated with me enough that I took it home to practice. Before this training, I was convinced that I wasn't doing it right and that I would never be able to do it. Not a lot has changed, except that I have given myself permission to do meditation badly, to fail at it over and over. The most important lesson I learned about meditation is that it is not a state of being zoned out; it is a state of being tuned in. It is noticing. It is letting go. It is finding internal space and spaciousness. We may not silence the monkey mind, but perhaps we slow it down.

I successfully practiced a daily meditation regime for a few months, and then my life changed significantly and I lost that sustained practice. I return to it again and again, in the spaces between sustained practice because I most certainly have noticed the benefits. The most effective meditation for me has been meditation focused on breathing, moving meditation, and meditation with mantras (usually a combination of all of these things). I have also found that taking embodied meditation-based classes, like yoga nidra, make it is easier to stay the course because I'm sharing space with other people who have committed to the practice. Many apps provide tools for meditation and for guided meditation. Insight Timer is a popular and prolific resource. It takes trial and error to find the meditation style that works for you, and to be kind to yourself when you feel like a failure. Already, you are doing yourself a favor by trying.

When I was teaching my Embodied Social Justice class in the spring of 2022, I found that I enjoyed writing guided meditations, and I had plenty of practice leading, or channeling, guided meditations in my work with women in recovery. For too long, I let one participant in the recovery program bully me into offering guided meditation every week because that was the yoga that she wanted to do. And, to be fair, it was summer and it was hot. But every time I tried to introduce something new, she would reject it and demand a guided meditation. As tedious and frustrating as this situation was, I greatly expanded my ability to improvise and innovate. Some of my favorite guided meditations play with the image, resonance, and metaphor of a tree or the colors and meanings of the chakras and their connections to the sacred elements of earth, air, fire, water, and ether. I continue to build upon these various approaches to meditation in my personal practice as well as my teaching, another ebb and flow that yoga offers. And sometimes meditation is resting my eyes and letting myself drift in that space between asleep and awake—a practice Tricia Hersey advocates for in *Rest Is Resistance*.

The Power of Mantra

While I find myself to be skeptical of many of the expectations of "positive thinking," there is something to be said for the power of the mantra. While mantras have a more specific and narrow meaning in traditional yoga, a mantra is simply a word or phrase that is repeated in the head or out loud, chanted or sung, alone or with other people. This repetition helps us focus and maybe even establish new patterns of thought.

In traditional yoga, mantras are in *Sanskrit*, the language of yoga, and these can easily be found through a variety of resources. The sounds of this language have resonance that we might feel even if we don't understand what the words mean. Some of these are primordial sounds that connect us to yoga's lineage and to our earliest ancestors. I prefer to use mantras in English because I am a mostly monolingual American asshole, but I have found resonance with some traditional mantras like *Om Namah Shivaya*. My favorite translation is "universal consciousness is one" and this is also described as a love song we sing to ourselves—fun stuff! And when we sing to ourselves, we are practicing self-soothing since the frequency of our voice is our own unique self-salve. Another mantra is *So Hum* ("I am") or just plain old *Om*, the vibration of the whole universe, universal consciousness, and a balance of body, mind, and spirit.

In Judith Lasater's book, *Living Your Yoga*, each chapter has a practice and a list of "Mantras for Daily Living." The mantras she includes are very much modern and in English. They fit with the theme of the chapter and the reminders and lessons we might need for living our yoga practice. For instance, in her chapter "Letting Go" she includes the mantras: "Detachment is the greatest act of love"; "I am willing to engage life"; and "This moment is the perfect moment to let go" (31).

In Gail Parker's book, *Transforming Ethnic and Race-Based Traumatic Stress with Yoga*, she includes a simple mantra as an affirmation to accompany each restorative yoga posture. For instance, in child's pose (*Balasana*) she suggests we repeat to ourselves: "Breathing in I feel innocent.... Breathing out I feel free" (41). Each chapter also includes a theme that she reflects upon and space to journal about the affirmation and how the practice benefits the reader. For instance, in the last chapter, "Birthing New Consciousness," she writes about the good and bad both being a part of life, about growth and loss, humiliation, disillusionment, post-traumatic growth, and healing narratives. She concludes with supported reclining bound angle pose (*Supta Baddha Konasana*) and suggests the practitioner repeat, "Breathing in, I feel whole.... Breathing out, I feel complete" (130). I love this book. I teach it in my Feminist Praxis for Radical Self and Community Care class, and I come back to it over and over.

I made use of mantras long before I realized what I was doing. On more than one hiking/backpacking trip, I have relied upon mantras to keep my feet moving (often through great pain—few of these are kind mantras!). A mantra distracts and focuses the mind simultaneously. It motivates and brings clarity of intention. A mantra should fit the person and the situation. And if you say it only in your mind, you are the only person who will know you are chanting a mantra. Match it to your breath (and movement) and—Boom!—meditation is happening.

Notice how mantras come to you spontaneously. Maybe you have a thought and an urge to repeat that thought. When you recognize a thought as a potential mantra, try repeating it. If it starts to hold power after you say it several times, play with it. Use it when you need it. Use it to replace negative self-talk. Create a ritual if you need it. Song lyrics make excellent mantras and there are plenty of classic yoga mantras set to music.

Here are some of my favorite mantras that sometimes fit and sometimes don't. They resonate in different ways at different times in different situations:

Interlude: Exploring Your Self and Embracing the "Woo-Woo" 59

- I am here in my body, in my body, in my mind
- Be kind in your thoughts; be kind in your intentions (said a yoga teacher in Denmark)
- I am grateful for all that I am. I am thankful for all that I have. I am humbled by all that I know. I am humbled by all that I don't know. I am grateful for the opportunity for more life, more love, more joy, more peace, more connection. I am.
- I am safe. I am grounded. I am centered. I am balanced.
- I am less than nothing. I am more than everything.
- My body, my mind, my beauty, my flow.
- And the classic: Be here now.

Something to Hold Onto

In meditation practice it can be helpful to have something to hold onto, something to connect to in a visceral, physical way. I have found that when I can connect with a physical object, I can better still my mind.

When I brought home my first stones, my ever-critical and neurologically-rigid husband said that they were for people with weak minds, people who needed to believe in some kind of magical force. I expected this rationalization even though I had not asked his opinion. When he said this, it made me wonder just how differently we individual human beings feel and experience the earth and the vibrations of energy in all things. Because, while I may not feel the powers ascribed to the rocks by the store's explanatory info cards, I certainly do feel something—something mostly indescribable. At the very least, a peace of mind. Maybe this is energy, or spirit, or imagination, or delusion. Ultimately, it does not matter. If a certain stone speaks to us, grounds us, eases our anxiety, who are we to judge the magic?

When I first went looking for some stones at my local Rock and Art Shop, I was looking for rocks that spoke to me. (I was also looking to find cheap rocks! There are many, many very beautiful and very expensive stones that spoke to me!) What I found was that the rocks that drew me visually also resonated with the ascribed qualities I was looking for. What speaks to us needs no deeper explanation than that which holds meaning for us. Some people can rattle off the particular properties of a stone, where it comes from, what it means. I cannot hold that level of detail in my brain and am always impressed when I meet someone who can. For some of us, we just know what feels right, and I have heard people describe powerful vibrations and other resonances from particular stones. Here are a few examples of stones that speak to me and help me to have something to hold onto in meditation practice or when I am over-worrying something:

- **Howlite**: reduces stress, anxiety, and tension. Encourages strength and expression, calms and soothes. Helps eliminate pain, stress, and anger.
- **Fire Agate**: associated with the essence of fire. Stabilizing, strengthening. Creativity and expression; sexual and physical energy, stamina, circulation, security, and self-confidence. Helps juggle commitments, write marketabley. Enables ability to take decisive action in unclear circumstances.
- **Olive Opal**: associated with the heart chakra. Healing and emotional purification, calming and protective, clarity and a relaxed mind. Emotional cleansing. Aids in relationships and a healthy diet. Balances mind, body, and spirit.
- **Pink Tourmaline**: focused on the heart to the crown. Love, joy, happiness. Emotional healing. Less stress and more ease and relaxation. Healing old wounds toward self-love. When found with some black: helps rid negative thoughts and relieve work stress. Works in challenging places and circumstances.
- **Botswana Agate**: balancing the emotional, physical, and intellectual.
- **Sun Jade**: mental organization and original thinking.

The stones above are generally colorful; those that follow are predominantly black, dark or reflective, mostly opaque:

- **Hematite**: absorbs negative energy; calms worry and stress.
- **Rhodonite**: heals emotional shock, scars, wounds; deep emotional peace.

- **Black Shiva** (South Indian origin): associated with the physical body and the lower chakras. Creativity, inspiration. Duality and universal consciousness. Balancing the masculine and feminine. A sex stone connecting to *kundalini* awakening. Stimulates energy flow throughout the body.
- **Guinea Fowl** (African origin): Associated with the liver, gallbladder, and stomach. Protects against negativity, grounding (root chakra). Gentle, relaxing, healing. Meditation, insight, creativity.
- **Apache Tear** (southwest U.S. origin): Heals grief. Protection, grounding.
- **Pyrite**: a stone of positive energy. Creates positive thinking and releases negativity. Brings about personal growth and success. Empowers the wearer to overcome anything.

*

Perhaps obviously, these stones can be worn as jewelry—bracelets, necklaces, pendants, etc. They can be something to gaze at, to hold onto, to decorate space—something to fidget, something to hold us together.

Oracle Cards

The more I have explored the woo-woo, the more woo-woo I have become. When I was taking my JourneyDance training, we started each session with about 20 minutes for personal practice. It was never enough time, but it was better than just sitting down to Zoom and jumping right in. The trainers encouraged us to set up stations around the room for different practices. One suggested practice was oracle cards. I hadn't used oracle cards before and I was skeptical. I had gone way out of my comfort zone a few years back when I finally became brave enough to change my life by changing myself. I had a Tarot reading done by my massage therapist and I found that it was far less woo-woo than I had imagined. It was like mental health therapy with props. Whatever magical or mystical qualities may be involved, the experience was a reading of cards in relationship to where I was in my life, what I wanted to know, and where I wanted to be. It was not that much different from what I do when I interpret a piece of literature or art. The Tarot reader uses her intuition to tell a story and the person getting the reading can take away the meanings that resonate with them. The reading told me a lot and helped to confirm the direction I was headed in, and when I came back to my notes and drawings from the reading a year later, I gained new insights.

So, when JourneyDance suggested Oracle cards, I thought: why not? At the very least, oracle cards are beautiful art and fun ideas to help us think in different ways and see things that we might not see in the normal course of considering our life and the universe. The practice of yoga, like the practice of using Oracle cards, can be frightening and threatening to some people. In my work with women in recovery, I found Oracle cards to be a way to settle the group and create opportunities for introspection, exploration, and hope. They loved the cards. Except, one day a new woman came to our yoga session and when I asked if she did yoga she told me, "No, I'm a Christian." That should have been a red flag that alerted me to introduce *The Wild Unknown Archetypes* deck by Kim Krans more delicately. But, I thought, archetypes are pretty universal and certainly a part of Christianity. She chose not to draw any cards, which is always just an invitation. As I read the descriptions from the guidebook to the other women, she became agitated and then announced that she doesn't agree with any of this as she stalked out. Lesson learned. I now take more time to explain the practice and connect it more directly to tools for self-reflection. I think of Oracle cards as being less threatening than Tarot, but they are clearly still a practice that can cause anxiety and disagreement.

Oracle cards are different from Tarot cards. Tarot has rituals and practices that vary, but has a long tradition in a variety of cultural contexts. Tarot cards have different ways of representing the major and minor arcana, but they are always the same 78 cards with minor variations like coins instead of pentacles or blades instead of swords. Oracle cards are unique sets of cards that are created by writers and artists and sometimes play off of the major and minor arcana of Tarot. Each has a theme and a guidebook with more information and different ways of doing readings, but the person using the cards can read them however they would like to read them. Nearly every time I have used them, the insights have been profound.

I suggest searching online for the cards that speak to you, or at a local store if you are so fortunate to have one near you. I'm a sucker so I initially bought three sets all at once. I already had a set of *The Sacred Self-Care Oracle* by Jill Pyle, beautifully illustrated by Tatiana Vedenkina, that I had not used before I started this practice. I vary which set I use depending upon my mood and what I feel intuitively from the cards on a particular day. Sometimes I choose the card that falls (or flies!) out of the deck. Other days I choose whatever feels right. One day I had my self-care cards laid out on a tapestry and my cat walked over them. One stuck to her foot and I decided to choose that one. It just happened to be the card that said spend time with animals. Yes, the universe is paying attention!

One of my favorite sets is *The Spiral Oracle* by Lili Acuña. Spirals resonate with me. I have been drawn to them my whole life and I have a couple different kinds of spirals inked on my body. They were an obvious choice. Each card is accompanied by a theme—like Alignment, Becoming World, Connection Link, Healing Path, I am, Inner Sun, Natural Abundance, The Journey (and many more)—and writings by the artist that does not seem to immediately match up with the theme of the card or the artwork, so I find many layered meanings in each one. I have only drawn the same card once and at first I was disappointed, but later I could see why I had drawn that card. My work with this deck is part of what inspired the name of The Spiral Goddess Collective, and my collection has grown (and continues to grow) as I include Oracle cards in my space and programs. When I brought this practice to my academic classes it grew to include social justice perspectives, informed and inspired by a project that one of my students did for another class and shared with me. Scholars like Hong-An (Ann) Wu and Caitlin (Catie) Lustig study tarot as a technology of care. Tarot is queered and interpreted through diverse cultural traditions by artists, activists, scholars, and practitioners.

My collection continues to grow. I have a *Mystic Martian Oracle* deck by Lisa Porter and *The Literary Witches Oracle* deck, written by Taisia Kitaiskaia and illustrated by Katy Horan (based on their book *Literary Witches: A Celebration of Magical Women Writers*).

These decks have two kinds of cards—extraterrestrial archetypes and sacred geometry linking cards in the *Martian* deck and the witches and the witches' materials in the *Literary Witches*—so they are fun to associate to each other and consider multiple possible interpretations. *The Wild Woman Oracle* by Cheyenne Zárate draws inspiration from the famous book *Women Who Run with the Wolves*. The copper, black, and white images are powerful and haunting. *The Dream Weaver's Oracle* by Colette Baron-Reid, illustrated by Joel Makamura, is quirky and colorful. The *Metaphysical Cannabis Oracle Deck* by Maggie Wilson, the first Black female cannabis sommelier (illustrated by Ejiwa Ebenebe), draws from African traditions, including plant medicine. This is a beautiful, multifaceted, and unique deck. It quickly became my new favorite. And then the *Magical Spirit Oracle* by Alexis Rakun, with 11 cards of each sacred element (earth, air, fire, and water), became my favorite. Now I have too many to pick favorites beyond a moment of engagement.

This is but a small sampling of the many different Oracle decks available. And, as it turns out, the deck that my massage therapist used was not actually a Tarot deck, but the *Dakini Oracle* deck, which is rare, but essentially the same as the *Tantric Dakini Oracle* deck that is now also a part of my collection and practice. In short, Oracle cards are a fun, intuitive, and creative way to continue self-exploration, regardless of how one feels about woo-woo. Some people might try to tell you that there is a right way and a wrong way to use Tarot or Oracle cards. At the 2023 Bangor Pride festival, The Spiral Goddess Collective had a vendor booth with a table full of inspiration for our work, including a few sets of Oracle cards. Several people explored the cards throughout the day. A few tried to walk away with the *Metaphysical Cannabis Oracle Deck*. A trans woman had a powerful reading about self-acceptance that brought her to grateful tears. Later in the day a woman came by with strong opinions about using cards, insisting that we had to pull three cards and that if we didn't we were putting a hex on her. We complied, and I'm still not sure if she thought she was doing a reading for us instead of us doing a reading for her. Like yoga, like all things, there is no one way to do anything. Rules are guidelines. We meet each experience, each yoga practice, each Oracle deck where we are.

Interlude: Exploring Your Self and Embracing the "Woo-Woo"

*

Maybe you find no woo-woo in this section. Perhaps you find woo-woo throughout this entire book. Maybe you love woo-woo! Perhaps any of this woo-woo opens you up to tap into imagination and the most unconventional insights about yoga that this book has to offer. But first, we have some things to unpack.

Two

Unpack

Perhaps we have found that blissed out yoga space where everything is rainbows and love and birds singing and stars zooming through a clear night sky. We feel the energy traveling the distance of our spine, our chakra's spinning in harmonic vibrations that mesh with the cosmos. Or something like that. And that's when there is this little voice at the back of the mind. The inner critic that stands ready to judge anything unfamiliar and also works hard to tear us down when we try something new. The guru might tell us that we need to silence that voice. It is a distraction. We are skeptical of the ease that others find, their ability to find blissful transcendence among chaos. Because we see contradictions, along with wishful thinking and blind acceptance, we find it difficult to take the good without focusing on the not-so-good.

We also see spaces and images dominated by thin, white, young, able (hetero)sexualized, female bodies. If we don't fit these images, or if we aren't able to fit in our bodies, we assume that these are spaces that are not open to us. Race, ethnicity, socioeconomic class, gender, sexuality, ability, religion/spiritual beliefs, geographical location, and nationality are key factors in how we experience the world and how we experience ourselves in the world, how we experience our bodies and minds in the world. And how we experience yoga.

*

All yoga experiences—even when we think these experiences are in the mind alone—are experienced in and through the body. And, vice versa, when we think that we are only doing yoga with our bodies, we are also engaging the mind and spirit. The language that peppers yoga classes may try to transcend the body and the baggage that bodies carry. But no matter how transcendent we may (try to) be, we are ultimately corporeal beings that are bound and gagged by the classed, raced, gendered bodies we inhabit. Further, we are these bodies in a world that grants and withholds material (and psychological) comforts based on these same categories. The lower we are on the hierarchies, the further from center we are at the intersections of race, class, gender, sexuality, and ability, the more likely our bodies/minds are to be devalued, dismissed, and destroyed.

We live in a segregated and stratified world. Maybe none of us feel normal even when we try our best to fit in. We feel like outsiders, misfits, interlopers, imposters. (And, spoiler alert: there is no such thing as normal!) Those with the privilege of fitting in while feeling things out may also feel uneasy in new spaces. Sometimes this is a function of unchecked privilege, but sometimes it is the demands of an inflexible set of social rules and expectations. Thus, we can't just make our interior spaces neater and less complicated, we also have to make the outside world more accepting and accommodating. This, too, is yoga.

If we are privileged to feel normal or to be seen as normal, we owe it to ourselves to think about how it must be to feel not normal and to challenge what is considered normal. We cannot solve the problems of power and privilege or change these conditions on (or maybe even through) our yoga mats. But we can at least be more aware of structural inequalities, more willing to embrace responsibilities that come with privilege, and more open to changing the material realities and misconceptions that contain Others, if only because they also contain us.

These conversations are bigger than most yoga studios can hope to touch upon, let alone grapple with. Such issues can't be sandwiched between postures and breath, but they cannot be ignored either. Some instructors, studios, websites, books, workshops, and spaces offer opportunities to engage with the social and cultural implications that manifest in the world despite yoga's positive vibrations. While the yoga world is beginning to try to be accountable to the realities of oppression and abuses of power, mixed messages and confusion abound. And many yoga practitioners might be able to ignore these bigger picture ramifications. (That privilege thing again!) At the very least, we can commit to staying curious and staying humble as well as staying open to negotiation of ideas and spaces.

Ultimately, there is no getting around contradiction and the social and cultural tension that comes with diversity. But we must not assume that contradiction is something to be gotten around. Instead, it is something to sit with. We can be blissed out in a moment and we can find our way back to that space when we need to. But we also have to be present in the realities that shape others' experiences of yoga and, thus, also shape our own experiences—the transcendent and the tragic. There is a difference between criticism and the art of being critical. Yoga often wants to see only the positive, but being critical—aware and conscious, observant and open—is necessary if yoga is to be anything more than exercise or personal mind/body/soul medicine. As we unpack the seedier sides of yoga, as we sift through the weeds and untangle the truths, we are forced to face complicated realities that don't mesh with the transcendent spaces and peaceful expectations associated with yoga.

Critique Is More Than Being Critical

I came to critical theory before I came to yoga. I came to yoga as a fitness instructor, and then as a student looking for healing, and always as a practitioner looking to share the benefits of my discoveries. Being a cultural critic shapes all of the things that I do, including teaching and practicing yoga. I learned from bell hooks: "I found a place of sanctuary in 'theorizing,' in making sense out of what was happening. I found a place where I could imagine possible futures, a place where life could be lived differently. This 'lived' experience of critical thinking, of reflection and analysis, [became] a place where I worked at explaining the hurt and making it go away" (*Teaching* 59). Critical theory and the consciousness it develops helps us explain the hurt and lessen it, and in this way critical theory is like yoga. Yoga is embodied critical consciousness. Cultural criticism (drawing from the tools of critical theory) is sometimes the best description of what I do, even if I am first and foremost a teacher. Cultural criticism and theory is one of the things I teach and this approach seeps from my academic teaching into fitness and yoga spaces. I bring my critical lens everywhere I go, and it is not always welcomed, especially in yoga spaces where being critical is often seen as being negative. But being critical is not about being judgmental or narrow-minded or abstract, it's about asking important questions, getting to root causes, exposing issues, reflecting and connecting, and as Jacoby Ballard notes in *A Queer Dharma*, "noticing gaps that need to be filled" (149). There are always gaps to be filled.

In my work in American studies, I have long practiced a central tenant of this field—that we have a responsibility to critique those things that we love. For instance, if we love our country, as so many patriotic (or not so patriotic) Americans do, then we have an extra responsibility to hold our country accountable to its principles and potential. Ballard makes this argument as well: "If I love something, I must be dedicated to its well-being and integrity" (195). It is our responsibility as yoga teachers, yoga practitioners, and as yoga participants to critique this thing that we love so much. It is also our responsibility as Americans to critique our country and as Americans who do yoga, we have the double layer of responsibility to critique American yoga in its various incarnations.

Positive Thinking

In some yoga spaces we want to turn to the promises of positive thinking. We assume that critique gets in the way of this easy answer. But, to move toward love, peace, and justice in our world, we need critique as much as we need positive thinking. Yoga can be an incubator for positive thinking theories. At its best, positive thinking reminds us that a good attitude and optimism can go a long way in helping us navigate life and its challenges. There is even some legit science that says that certain yoga techniques can help make us happier by boosting serotonin and releasing endorphins. Thinking positively can help our brains pay more attention to the positives in our lives. When we think positively, we have more control over how we react to the world around us, but we do not have control of the world.

Positive thinking cannot save the starving children, bring peace to the Middle East, or alleviate the bad behavior of entitled men.

There is certainly some truth and science to positive thinking; however, at its worst, positive thinking promises unearned riches and achievements as if such things can arrive out of thin air—from a vision board or a certain frequency of vibration. And at its most reprehensible, positive thinking blames the victim. This line of thinking precludes that people who have problems only have problems because of their negative thoughts, not because of a corrupt system or legacies of exploitation and unequal wealth distribution. This is the kind of thinking that promotes ideas like: people are poor because they don't work hard enough or racism only exists because Black people won't stop talking about it. But the reality is not so simple. Neither of these is true. Hard work does not automatically equal financial success; in fact, some of the hardest working people in our society fail to receive a living wage for their work (and are often working more than one job to try to make ends meet). And racism exists regardless of how much or how little we talk about it; it is structured into our institutions and it continues to shape our culture.

Oppression, positive thinking assumes, is a state of mind or a set of bad choices or a karmic punishment rather than a result of compounded ideologies, legacies, and policies. This is a dangerous effect (and affect) of "positive thinking," the kind of thinking that assumes the reality of power dynamics don't exist and that individuals—rather than systems and structures, traditions and institutions, unwritten rules and backroom power plays—are responsible for their bad luck in life. This is dangerous, uneven ground and yoga does not excuse us from our part in these systems. No matter how much "positive energy" we send out—as individuals or as collective groups—we still must live and act in a material reality where some people have a whole lot more than they need and some people have not even close to enough. Shifting the realities of systemic inequalities is a collective responsibility.

Not Yet Old Enough for Yoga

The prolific writer and social critic, Barbara Ehrenreich has written about the ways in which positive thinking has undermined progress in the 21st century. She has argued for the equity of the working classes. She has refused to be put through the rigors of modern medicine. She has challenged many partial truths and outmoded ideas. And for all her wisdom and insight regarding American culture and the body, she has also perpetuated ignorance around what yoga is. When I first read her book *Natural Causes* I expected an incisive analysis of the aging body in American culture (which she delivered); I did not expect a reiteration of yoga myths. She writes: "For a moment I even toyed with the ideas of a yoga class, possibly including meditation, before deciding that I'm not quite old enough for that" (69), and in her conclusion she notes that she "retain[s] a daily regimen of stretching, some of which might qualify as yoga" (207). Ehrenreich's discussion of yoga is mostly just disappointing. Here, a woman who has embraced the power and empowerment of weight lifting and the general health benefits of regular exercise, is so quick to dismiss yoga. She admits that she has pursued exercise, in part, to ward off aging and she vows that she is now old enough to die. And yet, she reduces yoga to something that is not worthy of her time.

Yoga has many relevant lines of inquiry toward her arguments and goals, even when yoga's ideas are abused as a means toward the impossible state of immortality. Yoga is not about trying to be younger or live longer—though some people might use it toward these ends. Instead, yoga improves the quality of life and the life of the mind. When respected public intellectuals like Ehrenreich perpetuate misunderstandings, we all suffer the consequences. I work with a lot of people who maintain the ideology that yoga is something for later in life, when they are old and cannot do the things they enjoyed doing in their more youthful days. However, when we practice yoga early and throughout our lives, it helps us to do the other activities we love and enhances our lives. Meditation has a range of physical, emotional, and mental benefits. Because yoga trains our bodies to retain our range of motion and our balance, for instance, it allows us to live with more independence as we age. We have better balance so we are less likely to fall and break a hip. We have range of motion so, as one yoga trainer phrased it, we can wipe our own butts. None of us can live forever; none of us can avoid disability or dependence on other people. These shallow ideas about age and yoga are directly connected to our cultural fixation on youth and our obsession with youth intertwines with our cultural obsession with Western ideals of beauty.

The Yoga Body (Beautiful)

The ideal of beauty—of strength, flexibility, acrobatic prowess, thinness, whiteness, and the "yoga body"—set impossible standards that make yoga seem inaccessible to most people. Almost every image we see online, in magazines, on television, and in brochures replicates the yoga body and its conventional beauty, if not also its incomprehensible bendability. The most beloved pop culture yoga figures are often also the most delicious eye candy, and celebrities who practice yoga are the prized examples of what yoga can do to sculpt a seemingly perfect body. This is an inherent aspect of American yoga; it is a side effect of superficial American culture, values, and expectations. We are a shallow culture, focused first and foremost on people's outward appearances and the power and influence that a beautiful appearance implies. This is only a statement of the obvious.

The tightly guarded yoga body is allowed some excess, some novelty, in the world of yoga personalities. My average body is too fat to be a "yoga body" but too thin to embrace "fat positivity." Big, magnanimous women are worshipped for their ability to perform yoga despite the size of their bodies while naturally thin women, riddled with eating orders, are praised for the beauty of their yoga bodies. Knowing I will never occupy either of these types of bodies, or their feats of strength and flexibility, is both comforting and endlessly frustrating. Letting go of the ways my body is judged and refusing to impose self-judgment is necessary, yet I am faced with its insidious nature more often than I would like to be. I don't like to be the center of attention, but I also don't like to be discounted. These feelings get in the way. At the same time that I seethe for a lack of recognition of my body as a yoga body, the instructor who looks like a stereotype seethes at herself, unable to see her own yoga body reflected back at her. We are all damaged by our cultural expectations.

In my teaching, in my very presence at the front of the room, I like to think that I am modeling that a fat body is also a yoga body, that a fat body is also a healthy body, a functional body, a beautiful body. And then I catch a glimpse in the mirror and wonder who that svelte woman is. She is certainly not me. And she is certainly not fat! And then, in that next glimpse, all I can see are the rolls of fat on my back, around my middle, and I am reminded that my body is not the body that is supposed to be teaching yoga. My personal hang ups and expectations about my body are a luxury and a privilege. I can imagine what it must be like to be a yoga teacher who fails to meet the stereotypes in more ways. And I can read about this experience online and in books and posts by people like Kimberly Dark, Anna Guest, Jessamyn Stanley, Teo Drake, Jacoby Ballard, Dianne Bondy, and many more. Many "brave" teachers break stereotypes and bring yoga to communities that need a model that looks like them. The Othered body, thus, becomes a starting point for a common practice that can be based on accepting difference despite ability. A focus on feeling and being and noticing instead of modeling feats of flexibility like the splits, or feats of strength like forearm balancing poses, can be one way to open up yoga spaces. When we value substance more than surfaces, when yoga is about going deeper within rather than showing off, we come closer to a yoga that is healthy and balanced and potentially transformative.

As much as I want to think of yoga as a welcoming space for all kinds of bodies, I can't help but notice that almost every yoga room I have been in has been dominated by the thin and white. I want yoga studios—and yoga spaces of all kinds—to be welcoming spaces, brave spaces, spaces for growth and rejuvenation. And it is not just the spaces that are unwelcoming; the bodies/minds that occupy these spaces are unwelcoming as well—to themselves as much as to others. Michelle Cassandra Johnson writes in *Skill in Action* that she "remember[s] being the only black girl in our [college] fitness class practicing yoga" and that her "understanding of oppression and privilege made [her] feel disembodied. That yoga class was not a space for affirmation, validation, or spiritual transformation" (xii). And it is not just racial difference that makes yoga spaces uncomfortable. Women who are afraid of being fat are afraid to take classes from instructors who model bodies that society deems as "fat" as if fat was contagious. People with disabled bodies who need support and options will not fit in yoga spaces. (And I think that we all need support and options!) Men and women and gender-fluid and gender non-conforming people who are anxious about the way they look or move, or their inability to be able to do something with their bodies—to stand out as different—tend to shy away from yoga studios. As Jacoby Ballard argues, "For trans people, our bodies haven't necessarily resonated with our identities or internal experiences of ourselves; to be told or invited to 'be in the body' when our bodies don't feel quite our own can feel naïve or cruel" (174). People who feel uncomfortable in their bodies for any number of reasons, including past experience or trauma, pain, or disability, fear yoga spaces. Changing this fact of yoga spaces is a start. Changing this fact of the larger culture is a related goal.

Yoga and Trauma

As we become more aware of the ways in which we are impacted by trauma—individually and collectively—we might hear the word trauma-informed or trauma-aware or trauma-conscious used to describe a yoga class or an approach to yoga. We might also hear about trauma-informed teaching practices in elementary schools or other settings. Soon, I hope, trauma-informed will be the approach to everything we do! When I opened The Spiral Goddess Collective, my founding vision was a trauma-informed space where all of the offerings would be informed by an awareness of trauma. I'm still working on shaping this reality, though we are far more aware than other yoga studios and spaces where yoga is offered. I also revised the "Integrated Healing Yoga" course for my university's nursing program so that it explicitly includes trauma-informed approaches and materials that address yoga and trauma explicitly. I have no interest in engaging with yoga that is not trauma-informed. And if nursing students are not studying a trauma-informed approach to understanding yoga, then we are doing a disservice to everyone they will come in contact with.

Trauma can result from any variety of experiences, and the same experience might result in trauma for one person but not another. The insidious thing about trauma is that its wounds run deep and its impacts can manifest themselves differently in every individual—in the mind and the body. There are common elements that span across different causes of trauma. Peter Levine, author of books like *Waking the Tiger*, describes trauma as any experience that overwhelms our ability to integrate it. As a result of trauma, we may suffer from post-traumatic stress (PTSD). Trauma, many studies have shown, is held in the body as much as in the mind. We might get it out of the mind, but if we don't get it out of the body, it will return and overwhelm. As I heard it phrased once: trauma gets under the skin. Or, the foundational phrase used widely: the issues are in the tissues. Trauma cannot be eradicated by talk-therapy alone because the physiological impacts of trauma are not logical, solvable problems. As Bessel van der Kolk's famous book title describes, the body keeps the score. There are many resources to explore that delve into this subject; we can find these resources when we are ready for them. Having an anchor or weaving a map of healing practices centered around breath and movement are powerful tools.

Many people are finding yoga techniques and spaces, teachers and communities, to be sources of healing. Trauma-informed trainings and community classes are becoming more common, and there is an array of books and websites devoted to these topics. The Justice Resource Institute and the Center for Trauma and Embodiment offer trainings in their TCTSY (Trauma Center Trauma Sensitive Yoga) program and the reach of trauma sensitive yoga classes is ever-expanding through such trainings. Nityda Gessel's Trauma-Conscious Yoga Institute offers her Trauma-Conscious Yoga Method and teacher trainings as well as workshops, webinars, on-demand classes, and a two and a half hour training called "Yoga for Social Justice: From Cultural Disembodiment to an Elevated Collective Consciousness." Gesell's book, *Embodied Self-Awakening: Somatic Practices for Trauma Healing and Spiritual Evolution*, extends her potential influence.

Overcoming Trauma Through Yoga: Reclaiming Your Body by David Emerson and Elizabeth Hopper offers a deep understanding of trauma and trauma-sensitive yoga as well as tips and techniques for survivors, teachers, and therapists. Arielle Schwartz's *Therapeutic Yoga for Trauma Recovery* mixes psychology and science with yoga practices, offering a map to individual, group, and therapy practices. Jamie Marich has some great tools in her book *Process Not Perfection*, which offers "expressive arts" activities toward processing and healing, many of which include breathing and movement techniques and a touch of yoga. Gail Parker addresses racial trauma specifically in her books. And while not specific to yoga, Resmaa Menakem's *My Grandmother's Hands* provides an important framework for understanding and working through race-based trauma. Many of the techniques he offers overlap with yoga practices.

Trauma is such an important topic generally, and specifically related to yoga, that I continue to connect to this topic throughout *Demystifying American Yoga*, starting in the next section, which explores one of the more difficult contexts related to trauma and later in this chapter in the section, "Trauma: From the Individual to the Collective." This might be a good time to reiterate that survivors of trauma should definitely seek help and insights beyond this book (beyond any book!). The help we find has to be help we're ready for. *Demystifying American Yoga* can be a start, a reminder that we are not alone (and we are not crazy or that we are and that's okay too) and that it is okay to get help with the things that are bigger than we are. Yoga teachers (as well as doctors, lawyers, educators, politicians, therapists, etc.) should understand the toll that trauma can take on the mind/body and how yoga—like life—can activate trauma responses.

Sexual Violence, Trauma, and Yoga

Unfortunately, the connections between sexual violence and the resulting trauma are insidious in our culture (and our world). Sexual violence is an umbrella term that encompasses the many ways in which bodies are used and abused by more powerful bodies, which includes the bodies of women and children, trans, femme, and non-binary folx, and men. All people can be victims—and survivors—of sexual violence (though patriarchal culture ensures that girls and women are more often impacted). And because trauma lives in the body, when we begin to move our bodies, even in the safest of spaces, we will inevitably encounter our trauma. As David Treleven writes, "Yoga is something of a double-edged sword when it comes to trauma. While many trauma survivors will benefit from yoga, the intense focus on sensations can also be dysregulating" (qtd. in Yamasaki xv). An understanding of how to teach in a trauma-informed manner is something that can make *everyone* feel more comfortable. This is especially important in yoga spaces where we are not only diving deep into our own bodies and minds, but we are also putting ourselves in spaces where we may encounter unwanted or unexpected touch.

I have been to many yoga classes where the instructor has not asked permission to touch people. I have been to yoga classes (mostly at conferences) where I've suddenly encountered "helpers" floating around the room making physical adjustments in addition to the instruction that is happening almost out of sight at the front of the room. I have been touched in ways that have made me uncomfortable, and I have been touched in ways that have forced me into a position of pain and physical distress. This experience makes me concerned for people who do not know that these things might happen in yoga classes. It makes me even more concerned for other survivors of sexual trauma, especially when we seek yoga as a form of, or alternative to, therapy.

Although I had read about and learned about the ways in which sexual assault might take place in a yoga class, I didn't fully understand what it might *feel* like until I experienced a particularly aggressive adjustment from an instructor in a yoga class on a college campus in Denmark. I saw her approach me and I expected her to touch me, but suddenly she slid her thigh between my legs from behind. She put her hands on my hips and pulled them back toward her body and then put one hand on my upper back. As she pushed me forward with the hand on my back, her abdomen and chest pressed firmly against my backside. She was like a flexible spoon. She pushed me past the physical limit of my flexibility. She could have pushed me beyond the limitations of my mental and emotional stability. If she had been a man, I most certainly would have been (re)traumatized. In the world of yoga, these kinds of adjustments happen all the time. Sometimes they are simply an aid to find a deeper pose. Sometimes they are calculated risks or instructors' habits, and they are often offered in good faith. Too often, they are predatory power moves. I have seen people shrink away from adjustments and I have seen people welcome them with a palpable hunger. Both responses to physical adjustments should be a call for pause and reflection. Both can be manifestations of trauma.

Another yoga experience brought out a trauma response from me that was unexpected. In my ongoing explorations of yoga, and for my academic research about yoga, I like to try out new yoga experiences. When I was teaching, living, and conducting research in Denmark, I decided to try out a free introduction to Tantric yoga. I didn't know what to expect. I knew that there may be sexual aspects, but I thought it was more about connecting with energy. I suspected there might be some uncomfortable moments. I dragged my husband along with me; he was willing to try out some new cultural experiences while we were on this grand adventure. When we were asked to participate in intimate poses with the partner we brought with us, I was already uncomfortable. I was uncomfortable for myself, but I was also uncomfortable for the other people in the room. One woman had come to this intro session solo, and the instructor did not do a good job of making her feel welcome. One couple was there for a "date night" experience (they were not dressed for yoga). One couple was young and had announced that they were there because they had attended a yoga class that was too athletic and intense, and they were looking for something more gentle. When they said this, I wanted to tell them that they were definitely in the wrong place. Later, I would have screamed it. But I remained silent; this was not my place to police.

I could handle the intimate yoga hug pose we did. When we were asked to form two circles, one with men on the inside and one with women on the outside, facing each other, I should have made a beeline for the door. Flight is what my body and mind told me to do. When the instructor asked us to gaze into our partner's eyes while we caressed them on the hands and arms, I could barely contain my desperate laughter, my shaking, and my tears. I did not know or understand at the time that I was having a trauma response, or that these feelings came from undiagnosed PTSD. I did not realize that I was in the middle of ongoing sexual trauma. All I knew was that my body was telling my mind to run away. My mind was spinning and telling my body I had no choice but to stay. And then she told us to take a step to our right and to do the same exercise with another person—with another man, with a stranger. I don't know how I survived. I felt like an adolescent girl with uncontrollable giggles and I swallowed these reactions as best I could. I pretended to be okay. I was sure that everyone could see that I was definitely not okay.

I felt violated and betrayed. I think I survived because I could objectively critique the many horrible qualities of this yoga workshop. I stood outside of myself at that moment. I could laugh about it afterwards, sharing the experience with other Americans, and pretending that it did not shake me to my very core. It was only one of many difficult and uncomfortable experiences that came with living in a different culture and a different country; I bundled it with those other more benign experiences. I soon started teaching my own brand of yoga in Denmark and could compose myself enough to survive the rest of my stay. Moreover, I could heal just a little bit by offering a different kind of yoga experience to the people who took my classes.

*

While yoga can be a healing therapy after traumatic experiences, yoga can also be the source of a new or renewed trauma. In the #MeToo era, yoga has not been immune to criticism or the stories of victims and survivors and many yoga organizations have responded to the #MeToo movement with additional resources and interventions. There are too many stories of mostly women who have been taken advantage of by mostly male teachers. I imagine that these men have large egos and the ability to insulate and disillusion themselves with their power and influence. This is exactly the story of Bikram Choudhury and too many others. Obviously, women can exploit this power too. They can prey on students who might have assumed that they were safe with a woman in ways that they could not feel safe with a man. I imagine that many of the women who fall prey to yoga-teacher predators have been absorbed into their charisma. But there are many variations on sexual assault—all violations of bodies and minds, trust and vulnerability.

Through Nityda Gessel's mailing list I was introduced to Zahabiyah A. Yamasaki's work as the founder of Transcending Sexual Trauma through Yoga (an organization that offers trauma-informed yoga to survivors as well as consultation for universities and trauma agencies, and training for healing professionals) and her book, *Trauma-Informed Yoga for Survivors of Sexual Assault: Practices for Healing and Teaching with Compassion*. Gessel and Yamasaki offer a yoga training program package that combines their work. Yamasaki's work is also made available through a trauma-informed yoga affirmation card deck, illustrated by Evelyn Rosario Andry, a companion to her book. The cards offer "a holistic healing process" and "supportive and compassionate guidance for survivors of sexual assault" through affirmations paired with trauma-informed yoga practices that are explained and illustrated on each card. Yamasaki's book is a rich resource for healing one's own trauma as well as working with survivors on their healing paths. In "A Note Amid the Pandemic," Yamasaki writes:

> This book is a combination of personal narrative, survivor truths, supportive guide for those passionate about trauma-informed yoga, fierce yet tender lens of advocacy, and soft place to land for survivors. I always say that **showing up is the hardest part**. So I invite you to take a moment to send yourself compassion for everything it took to get to this very moment.... I hope this book can be a healing balm, a place of refuge and retreat, and a container for all you may be holding. Thank you for trusting and traveling this journey with me. It is an honor to have you hold this book in your hands and your hearts [xiii, author's emphasis].

What follows is a lot of love, science, research, personal and professional experience, resources, tools, guidance, support, and so much more.

Yoga has been key to my own healing of trauma, and the books and teachers I cite offer new perspectives, practices, tools, comrades, and communities. Through my teaching, in academia and through yoga, I try to create opportunities for people in my community to learn more about trauma—and more about tools for addressing trauma in the body. I am still carving my own path through the wilderness, toward healing and perhaps beyond.

Integrating Binaries

Yoga, as previously noted, means union. And Hatha yoga is a union of sun (*ha*) and moon (*tha*)—the power of opposites pushing against each other to create stability. There are many binaries that arise in life and in yoga: masculine/feminine, self/other, right/left, right brain/left brain, reason/intuition, ancient/modern, universal/particular, conscious/unconscious, fire/water, East/West, physical/spiritual, traditional/revolutionary. In many cultures we assign masculine and feminine meanings to these binaries where the sun, for instance, is active and powerful and the moon is receptive and weak. In yoga, these opposites are not resolved or overcome; they are held in creative tension. They are paradoxically integrated. They are both/and instead of either/or. In yoga there is wholeness and integration even though some practices reinforce the binary.

These lessons of integration can be practiced through yoga poses that help us to engage the right and left brain and poses that help us to coordinate the right and left sides of our bodies. For instance, spinal balance treats both the physical and the mental senses of balance. Through the art of paying attention, we can also notice the ways in which the sides of our bodies are different—one hip tighter than the other, for instance. We are built asymmetrically. More, yoga can help us to reflect upon the imbalances in our thoughts and emotions. We can notice anxiety and calm it with a slower breath, extending our exhale. We can notice depression and lift it by opening our chest and finding an equal ratio to our deep belly breath. We can balance our sympathetic and parasympathetic nervous systems.

We can also use yoga to practice the difference between thinking and feeling. We can get out of our heads and into our bodies. We can contemplate a problem endlessly and find no solutions, and then we can move through it with our breath coordinated with our movements and the very problem has been transformed. In poses, we might find a balance between thinking and feeling. We might pay attention to a variety of alignment cues that we are given as we sink into warrior II; and/or, we might notice what it feels like in our body and our mind as we sink into warrior II pose. We can interrupt the kinds of movements that create muscle memory and lock us into certain planes of antagonistic motion as well as rigid ways of thinking. We can change our bodies by changing our minds and change our minds by changing our bodies. Circles and figure-eight motions can also help us break binaries as we shift out of the linear movements that we are often conditioned to embrace. We can become more flexible thinkers, creating new pathways in our brains through novel movement.

Yoga helps us to embrace the now and to balance the binaries of past/present and present/future. When we find our minds wandering to the past, the sensation of our breath can bring us back to the present moment. When we find ourselves worrying about the future, feeling our feet on the earth can bring us back to the present through the sensations in our body. These are some of the ways that contradictions are embodied and moved into non-binary states. Perhaps yoga can also help us unpack the black/white binary of race in the U.S. But maybe even yoga isn't that powerful!

Unpacking White Supremacy

White-bodied people (a term used by Resmaa Menakem) have to accept and understand that white people and ideologies of individualism, perfectionism, elitism, imperialism, and objectivity, for instance, have caused harm in our world over and over again. Individual and institutional acts of racism, sexism, classism, and more, have divided and conquered, exploited and murdered individuals, groups, and communities. This is an understatement. American culture is a culture of white supremacy, overlapping with what Tricia Hersey calls grind culture. This culture impacts all of us negatively, creating unrealistic expectations for ourselves and others. White people need to take responsibility to help stop these toxic cycles, but we don't have to take on the shame and blame. Unfortunately, too many of us are in denial, at best, and in aggressive opposition at worst.

In writing about the critique that his co-founded Third Root Community Health Center received, Jacoby Ballard notes that "we absorbed the critiques that had been waiting in the wings after so many institutions had just not been able to hear them" (200). Throughout my career, I have absorbed many critiques of the work I do, in and out of academia, earned and unearned. Sometimes white people doing the work of social justice face critique for simply being white-bodied in a world that has been dominated by white-bodied people and principles and practices of white supremacy. I get it. I have beat myself up at times for daring to do the work that I do, for taking up space that could, or should, be filled by someone with a more fitting identity, someone who has navigated the racism and/or homophobia that my physical appearance protects me from. My first job interview as a Ph.D. student was for a position as a professor of African American studies in an ethnic studies department. On paper (and on the phone) I was more than qualified; in person, I was not what the students were looking for. I was not what the administration was looking for. They both wanted a Black body, but for different reasons. The students wanted and needed a mentor. The administration wanted and needed a token. Both assumed that a Black body could (and should) meet this demand. During the campus visit, I was put in the impossible position of arguing for why I should be hired for a job that I wanted—and knew I could do—but I didn't think I should have.

At the end of the two-day campus interview process, I lunched with the (white) chair of the department and we chatted informally. I mentioned that I was a yoga teacher and I could see the look on her face as she hammered the last nail in my coffin. The fact that I was white was one thing; the fact that I was white *and* I taught yoga signaled that I was *one of those* white people. Lesson learned. Unfortunately, this lesson caused a separation between my mind and body and undercut what was already a tenuous hold on confidence. My career in academia wanted only my mind while my "hobby" (my lifeline, my passion) wanted only my body. I toggled between the two and often tore myself apart. Yoga, and embodied movement through conscious dance, put me back together.

So many institutions, so many people in power still can't hear the critiques—or even the cries—of the most oppressed and marginalized members of our society. We have not yet worked through our collective cultural trauma. We have not transformed harmful systems and structures. We have not yet reached that magical historical/cultural moment where we can trust that a white person is not going to default to privilege and unearned power when the going gets tough. We cannot "just get along" or be judged on the "content of our character"; in fact, we mock and manipulate these famous sentiments as we blame the victims. Too many white people refuse to hear or see the truth of Other experiences. Too many Othered people cannot see past their own pain. In both cases, "some people may not have healed or are in a cycle of rage or grief that prevents connection" (110), as Jacoby Ballard explains. This is where we circle back to yoga.

Ballard challenges the common notion in yoga social justice circles that we need to bring yoga to "'those who need the practice most,' which often implies low-income communities, communities of color, and other communities with high incidences of trauma" (183). I have fallen into this sentiment even as I internally struggled with the idea and feeling that "we all need healing, and we all deserve it" (183). Further, I have wondered what impact yoga and critical consciousness combined might have on those who have power and privilege and "how impactful these practices [mindfulness, meditation, yoga] could be for those holding the most power in our world, if they contemplated and acted from their inherent connection, rather than imagined separation" (183). We all need yoga. We all need more tools for self-regulation, compassion, empathy, and connection. As Gail Parker argues, "Regardless of race and ethnicity, we are all impacted by its damaging effects, from those who are wounded to those who intentionally or unwittingly do the wounding" (*Transforming* 19). Our culture breeds hurt, isolation, shame, inadequacy, comparison, and disconnection. We are all hurting.

The amount of our pain is not a competition, but it is a call for concern and an opportunity for healing. Pain plus power is a recipe for disaster. It is the recipe that contributes to mass shootings, patriarchal violence, and hoarding, for instance. Jacoby Ballard argues that "when we understand that 'hurt people hurt people,' the healing of wealthy people, men, white people, and others with privilege is absolutely necessary, alongside those in positions of privilege reckoning with the wreckage caused in its wake" (187). Imagine what this would mean for American culture, society, and institutions—let alone individuals—who do great harm from often unrecognized places of hurt. If Donald Trump had had a loving mother and a generous grandfather, if he had been taught breathwork and self-regulation (yoga!) at an early age, if he had been taught that his family's wealth and power came with responsibility to make the world a better place rather than an excuse to lie, cheat, manipulate and exploit, would he wreak such havoc? Maybe, but probably not. Trump embodies the most extreme version of white privilege and his narcissism trickles down to the masses of (mostly white) mostly men who are hurt and hurting. Closer to home interventions that provide opportunities to confront, process, and heal white men's real and perceived hurts might just have the power of grassroots organizing and bottom-up transformation. And white women who bolster and placate these men, out of choice or survival, are implicated as well. All of us need to unpack white supremacy.

Not only do "hurt people hurt people"; perhaps more importantly, hurt people help people and hurt people *heal* people. Hurt people who engage in healing practices, in community and through the internal work that yoga can foster, help to heal other hurt people—as practitioners of healing arts and as models of what Ballard calls "vicarious resilience." Opportunities for the positive impacts of healing come on the heels of our critiques of systems and structures that serve none of us and hurt all of us. Yoga, as it has grown and festered in mainstream American culture, also needs to be critiqued and transformed to better serve the healing salve that yoga provides.

Pretty Fly for a White Girl

Did I mention that I am white? It cannot escape our attention that yoga in America has been largely practiced, purchased, defined, and shaped by white women, specifically white women with class privilege and heterosexual cisgender privilege. This is not the whole story or the whole picture, but it does explain some of the reasons why American yoga has been narrow, damaging, and exclusive. American women are really good at drinking the Kool-Aid. We embrace and embody damaging cultural narratives and we spread these ideologies even when they hurt us directly. White women are especially guilty of engaging in unconscious consumption of yoga—and many other cultural practices, symbols, and products. Sell it to me on a trendy t-shirt and I will wear it with self-righteousness!

Yoga can't be just another trend, another exercise regime, another promise of aging gracefully. It can't be expensive and exclusive. It can't be Karen's comfort zone. It can't be about accessories or gatekeeping. White women with good intentions cannot escape this cultural trap. But we can all put in work—on ourselves, first and foremost, and on the larger culture of American yoga where we compete and consume. We must go below our surface expectations and anxieties as much as we must go beyond yoga's surfaces. We must change our paradigms.

White women who teach yoga (like me!) have the most work to do. We have the most responsibility because we have taken the most. This idea used to rankle me. I was upset that my teaching of yoga, in and of itself, could be offensive. I avoided the elements of yoga that felt inauthentic in my teaching and thought I would be safe from the traps of cultural appropriation if I stuck to a fitness-based yoga. The avoidance of appearing to appropriate led to a hollowed-out practice and this avoidance became impossible (and less desirable) the further I journeyed into yoga trainings, teachings, and practices that look nothing like "fitness." Or rather, teachings and practices that shifted the meaning and practice of "fitness" have transformed the way I approach my yoga and fitness teaching as well as my personal practices. In embracing my whole self and attempting to align my yoga teaching as part and parcel with my academic teaching about embodiment, intersectionality, and social justice, I have found deeper meaning and renewed passion. While I continue to learn, evolve, and grow in and through this work, it is never easy. My academic background shortened the learning curve for imagining how yoga might be a tool toward social justice. We all must make this journey, but we might get there via different paths and at different paces.

Ultimately the onus is on white people—the group with the most power and privilege—to, as Susanna Barkataki argues, "create diverse [and inclusive] spaces"; "to learn from, uplift and share the many faces of ancient and modern wisdom"; and to "hear from the indigenous knowledge-keepers and way-showers of yoga today" (9). This is a tall, but necessary, task that begins with humility and empathy. Barkataki points out: "South Asians and Desis (*Desis* is a term for diasporic Indians who live outside India) are actively excluded from positions of leadership in yoga" (89). This is a problem that she has begun to rectify through activism, writing, and creating her own brand of yoga teacher training. Supporting leaders like Barkataki and other yoga teachers with ancestral connections is important, but tokenism is not the answer. As Ballard points out, "exoticization of South Asian teachers that presumes their wisdom based on their identity rather than their practice" (140) is also problematic. There are examples of individuals who come from a place (like India) and teach yoga in the U.S., not because they have studied yoga as a part of their life, upbringing, and culture, but because their identity becomes their credential. We (white yoga teachers, studio owners, and practitioners) are sometimes too afraid of being perceived as racist to hold Indian/South Asian teachers, let alone teachers of color more generally, to the same standards as we hold white teachers. (And, in some spaces and cases, we might also fail to hold yoga teachers to any standard at all!) This racist dynamic is a problem in and out of yoga spaces.

The body we teach from is the point from which assumptions are made (and body size, rather than racial or ethnic identity, is probably where the initial judgment is made!). White people who teach yoga, or Black people who teach yoga, or anyone who teaches yoga, are authentic when our teaching is based upon our *practice* and study rather than our (perceived) identity. Our practices of yoga are diverse and based upon many different training models, teacher trainings, and yoga schools in the U.S. What each of us brings to our own teaching is not based solely upon our categories of identity.

Identity in the U.S. is complicated, but the larger structures of white supremacy still shape the way we see and are seen in the world and in the world of yoga. It only follows that the way we practice would also be shaped by white supremacy, patriarchy, and capitalism. Entangled in isms, there is more to unpack.

Objectification, Exoticism, and Cultural Appropriation

Yoga crosses many cultures that have transformed the practice across time and space. In fact, yoga's transformation over time has been shaped by forces of all kinds—political, economic, spiritual. Individuals and social movements, corrupt and/or transformative, have tapped into the power of yoga in India and in the U.S. (and in other places). As Susan Raffo argues, "When healing traditions shift from one cultural tradition to another, they continue to evolve and shift" (201). While it is impossible (and, perhaps, undesirable) to distill the original experience of yoga into something authentic in 21st-century America, a healthy respect for cultural origins can go a long way. In other words, adorning bodies in mandalas and Ganesh t-shirts, decorating spaces with statues of Buddha and Hindu goddesses, and using singing bowls and chanting (not to mention the physical postures themselves) should not be done without some consciousness and respect. But who decides what a healthy dose of respect entails and what infringes upon the sanctity of a practice or a symbol? What amount of reverence counteracts appropriation? For instance, if I close a class with *Namaste* (an Indian greeting appropriated as a closing sentiment in many yoga classes), I feel uncomfortable, but if I don't, I feel disrespectful. Participants have come to expect a *Namaste* to close a class, so much so that if I say something different in closing, they still say *Namaste* in answer.

Cultural appropriation is even more convoluted by the rise of exotic yoga retreats in places like Bali and Costa Rica. These retreats are located in places where yoga has become one more cultural commodity among tiki torches and poolside bars. They are often seen as more authentic (or maybe just more desirable) simply because their locations are more exotic than U.S. locations. The location promises relaxation and rejuvenation at least as much as the yoga that will take place there. Many people travel to India in order to get a taste of authenticity and some American yoga teachers train, or supplement their training, in India. Some American teacher trainings or individual teachers create partnerships with Indian yoga teachers and schools. Certainly, some yoga experiences in India, or taught by Indians in the U.S., are shaped by and for American expectations. Further, yoga's roots in ancient India are complicated by similar spiritual practices in China and Africa, for instance, or by indigenous practices around the world. How many times have ancient practices been borrowed and bent? Who owns spirituality, for instance? If a spiritual practice from another culture resonates with someone from a different culture, who determines whether this person is allowed to take up an indigenous spiritual practice (or a variety of practices) as their own? And American spiritual explorations are not new. As Stanley notes in her chapter from *Yoke*, "Cultural Appropriation Is More American Than Apple Pie," "Since before the nineteenth century, White yoga practitioners can be found making their way to and from India and other Asian countries on spiritual pilgrimages as a way of claiming a deeper connection to their own spirituality" (97).

There are many conversations—in yoga spaces, in academic spaces, in online spaces—that debate issues of cultural appropriation and there are no steadfast answers. One thing that is consistent in discussions of cultural appropriation is the role of power and exploitation or the stake of profit. Many people in these conversations agree that if someone is using a cultural tradition (yoga, cacao ceremonies, or sweat lodges, for instance) in capitalistic practice, if they are profiting off of traditions that have origins and meaning in other cultures and not citing or compensating the people from those cultures, particularly traditionally oppressed cultures, then they are engaging in a form of cultural appropriation that does damage. I do not disagree, but appropriation is far more complicated. The line is not so easy to draw, though some examples are so egregious that no debate is necessary.

We all need to make a living in this system we have not chosen. Yoga in America has empowered many women to open small businesses. These small businesses help them to be financially independent (when they don't fail miserably or make barely enough to cover their costs, which is often the case with yoga or fitness studios) and can also help them empower other women in their communities. Are they "wrong" for making a living from the cultural practices that originate in non–Western parts of the world? Are they wrong only if profit outpaces a particular threshold? Is it okay if they are non-profit? They were trained and sanctioned by schools of yoga that have created a product to sell to individuals who pay a lot of money for the privilege of making a living (or trying to make a living). Is this where the wrongness begins? These schools pay to be certified and are held to a set of standards determined by Yoga Alliance, and who crowned Yoga Alliance with such powers? All these players are profiting off of yoga and producing further streams of potential profit, appropriation, and exploitation. In some places, people and institutions have stopped offering *yoga* classes, changing the name of the classes from yoga to something benign, like stretching. Part of this conversation is about respect. Part of it is about power. It is a vicious cycle with no easy answers. If we call it "mindful stretching," is this better? Or worse?

As I shared in my book, *Women and Fitness in American Culture*, in graduate school a colleague (originally from Bangladesh) shamed and mocked me during a departmental meeting for teaching yoga at the campus fitness center. I was a student, a teaching assistant, and none of my other colleagues defended me, some of whom were people of color (who were not Indian) who regularly attended yoga classes. And he was not wrong about my ignorance at that point in my training. But his words stung, mostly because they were delivered with condescension and derision and he used his race/ethnicity, and not his yoga *practice*, as his barb. At the time, I was not confident enough to defend myself. Part of this lack of confidence came from my lack of training, and part of it came from the white guilt that weighed heavily on me at that point in my still-developing career path. Maybe I deserved to be called out; maybe we all need to be humbled. But who appoints the judge? Who instructs the jury? Who doles out the punishment? Who gets the last word? Stanley's chapter sheds much light. She notes that "maybe there's an imperialist in all of us" (108). She reminds us that "avoiding cultural appropriation means exploring the reasons why we appropriate. Inevitably, it means gazing upon and accepting the colonizer inside of you. This self-exploration is yoga in action" (104).

*

For a long time, some British scholars refused to accept the legitimacy of *American* literature; to them, it was only a watered down derivative of the original product—British literature which is really only Literature. As Dianne Bondy notes, the Western influence on yoga can be seen "through many accessible yoga modalities as well as the development of fitness-centered yoga." Is it possible that *American yoga* is its own thing? Has it outgrown the prescriptions of its parent culture(s)? Maybe. If so, our critical vigilance is all the more important. Asking how we can "teach practices ... that build collective power, collective accountability, and help to heal our collective bodies as well as our individual ones" (201) is a question that Susan Raffo asks us to grapple with. The "collective liberation" that Raffo writes about calls for a deeper dive into what diversity looks like (and how it functions) in yoga spaces.

Diversifying Yoga

The work of diversifying yoga requires a critical lens that goes beyond the reductionist idea that diversity is about, as Barkataki argues, "tak[ing] a tally of who is there and who is not" (133), an argument that is echoed by other people who write about yoga and diversity. The aspects of our identity that contribute to diverse yoga spaces and practices are not always visible when we look around yoga spaces, particular yoga *studios*. Only the most superficial aspects of diversity are visible, though we might also argue that these superficial aspects (skin color, hair texture, eye shape) are also the most likely targets of oppression. Our *consciousness* of our racial identity very much shapes how we come to yoga and conversations about yoga, and racial identity intersects with other aspects of our identity like gender, sexuality, ability, nationality, and more. Diversity as a dimension of whiteness is often lost in discussions about diversity and inclusion as well as race and social justice. Where and how white people (and Black people, and all people) enter the conversation and practices of yoga, and how we learn to "properly embrace [our] practice" (Barkataki 6), is worth a deeper dive and a critical eye. When we tease out the intersectionality of oppressed (and privileged!) groups, what else might we find?

When addressing her generic reader in *Embrace Yoga's Roots*, Barkataki is sometimes explicitly addressing white people as a monolithic category of yoga teachers and practitioners separate from all other racial/ethnic categories. Toward the end of the introduction she instructs "you" her generic reader to explore and "examine the social norms and constructs that you've helped erect in yoga in the West" (18). Perhaps perpetuate is a better word than erect; the social norms of "yoga in the West" were *erected* long before many of us starting practicing. These are the same norms as American culture more generally (Tatum's smog in the air), which makes them largely invisible to mainstream Americans; and, whether visible or not, these norms shape the experiences and ideas of all Americans regardless of race, in and beyond yoga spaces. American yoga lacks a consciousness of these social and cultural norms and, by extension, lacks a consciousness of yoga's historical and cultural roots. Embracing yoga's *roots* is Barkataki's focus; and in making her arguments, she sometimes misses the nuances of America's cultural landscape.

Barkataki is patient with her audience of yogis. She encourages the reader to meet the material in her book where they are. She empathetically cautions: "if you find yourself triggered then take care of yourself and continue to re-engage" (18). She reminds us that "this work is continuous and ever-evolving" (18). She notes that "you may respond differently depending upon your positionality. Whether you are South Asian, Black, Indigenous, Person of Color or white" (7). Certainly racial and ethnic identity influences how we read Barkataki's book, as well as how we practice and teach yoga. But is racial "positionality" the defining factor? At one point, in a very short section about "Yogis and Intersectionality," she notes: "Again, this doesn't mean don't practice or teach if you aren't Indian. It does mean lifting up your BIPOC, South Asian and Indian counterparts" (172). However, just because white people dominate mainstream

American yoga and perpetuate social norms and constructs erected decades ago, doesn't mean that all white people are in a position to do the lifting up. Barkataki's argument lacks an intersectional understanding of whiteness, assuming that American yoga spaces are only what we see in the dominant, mainstream media and yoga culture.

Jacoby Ballard extends and clarifies this argument, noting that "we must commit ourselves to consistent and never-ending study and being honest about our training ... and give opportunities to skilled teachers not yet in the spotlight, with special attention to those from marginalized communities" (200). Ballard's focus on "opportunities" and "special attention to those from marginalized communities" speaks to American diversity. This might look like the spotlighting that Jivana Heyman offers in his book through interstitial boxes that capture the voice, practice, and approach of diverse yoga teachers. "Special attention to those from marginalized communities," is something that any of us can do as we teach and share the wisdom upon which we have built our practice and pedagogy and marginalized communities are intersectional communities that are not always defined along racial lines. Ballard argues, "writing about this dynamic and my benefitting from it is the least I can do" (135). But it is not the least they do. Ballard also pays reparations, lifts up teachers with different marginalized identities, aims for generosity, gratitude, and humility, pursues continuing education, and offers critiques of mainstream yoga that call us all in. Ballard models what diversification (and decolonization) of yoga looks like from a white body.

*

In social justice circles, we lump people from racialized marginalized groups together under the category of BIPOC, and segregate these groups from white, sometimes without awareness or explanation of why BIPOC is afforded special status (because of shared histories of oppression). In doing so, we also erase complexity and intersectionality. Writing for a U.S. audience in her book, Barkataki includes BIPOC in the same category as South Asians and Indians, setting white people aside as the ones who need to lift up nearly everyone else. At the same time, she argues that yoga's roots are South Asian and Indian and she defends these boundaries as she encourages her reader to embrace this particular history, to pay homage and to center contemporary South Asian practitioners.

Barkataki's arguments make a leap that many readers may not follow. We might argue, along the lines of the responsibility that comes with privilege and access, that white people should lift up our BIPOC counterparts because they are marginalized within the larger systems and structures, histories and landscapes of U.S. racial politics. Whiteness has dominated American institutions that need to be diversified (or dismantled and rebuilt); American Yoga also needs to be diversified (and, perhaps, dismantled and rebuilt). This might be the unstated assumption that Barkataki is working within because she does not make an argument, like Dianne Bondy in "The Black History of Yoga," that "there may be multiple cultural sources in different geographical locations that created their own yoga traditions of mindful-movement practices ['whether in the form of dance, asana (postures), or exercise']." For Barkataki, there is only one yoga, which was "legally and de facto banned in India under British rule and colonization," resulting in lost lineages and thousand-year-old traditions ("How to"). These banned practices, she argues, are the same practices that "millions of Westerners now turn to for alternative health and wellness therapies" ("How to"). This history of colonization by the British in India most certainly seeps into American contexts, but we can't necessarily draw a direct line. Yoga's influence meanders.

When she uses the term BIPOC, Barkataki does not argue, for instance, that Black Americans do, in fact, have a connection to yoga's roots that may be older than yoga's roots in India. To be fair, very few people in the world(s) of yoga make this argument, which might be because of those larger cultural trends of erasure of Black people and Black histories, in the U.S. and around the world. (Bondy makes a similar argument.) Barkataki, and many other people writing about diversity, cultural appropriation, decolonization, and social justice in (and beyond) yoga spaces gloss over other possible roots of yoga. Perhaps embracing yoga's roots calls for us to cast a wider net and take a deeper dive. Dianne Bondy argues that yoga's "origins are likely far richer and more complex." Harnessing the power of yoga toward individual and structural healing and transformation means embracing yoga's deep and wide roots.

Yirser Ra Hotep illustrates how "the people of ancient Kemet practiced a unique style of Yoga that predates the Yoga of India, and the practice and philosophy of Yoga in India was informed by knowledge that came out of Africa." He argues that "the Yoga of Egypt is much older than that found in India." We really can't know the multifaceted origins of contemporary yoga, but we can recognize that African roots and American roots are part of yoga's long history—whether they are origins or parallel practices. Further, we can embrace a multiplicity alongside critique of "the power imbalance that remains between those who have access to wealth, an audience and privilege in contrast to those who have been historically marginalized" (Barkataki, "How to"). Ultimately, the power imbalance, not identity, can be the target of social justice. Identity is multifaceted; power imbalance, while insidious and wide-ranging, is easier to map.

Kemetic Yoga has roots in Egypt, but we might argue that it is a form of *American* yoga as "The modern version of this ancient system was developed from primary research conducted by Dr. Asar Hapi and Master Yirser Ra Hotep (Elvrid Lawrence) of Chicago during the 1970s." Kemetic yoga had to be rediscovered and reimagined, like all things lost to dominant, white, patriarchal histories. The 1970s was a prime time for cultural excavation; scholars and activists continue to do this work. Yoga's roots in Egypt were lost long before yoga came to the U.S., and before British colonization of India. Reclaiming and building foundations for these ancient, rooted practices happens in (and beyond) U.S. contexts, diversifying American yoga alongside Indian yoga. Hotep created Kemetic YogaSkills, which includes a 200-hour Teacher Training and Certification sanctioned by Yoga Alliance. As Dianne Bondy notes, "Reading about the connections between Africa and yoga has reaffirmed for me that the practice is in my blood, that I fit into this culture." Bondy's "fit" illustrates one of the ways we can "lift up" Black American yoga teachers and practitioners as connected to yoga's ancient roots, rather than as a part of the BIPOC language of social justice. Further, the Black Yoga Teachers Alliance, founded in 2009, continues to grow and shape the American world of yoga and their list of partners and sponsors reflect the support of big business (like lululemon) as well as industry leaders (like Kripalu).

*

Barkataki's focus is not on diversifying so much as *decolonizing*, which is an approach that cannot be carried out solely on the individual level. However, we can certainly take steps to individually decolonize our practice and Barkataki guides the reader through some advice in, "How to Decolonize Your Yoga Practice," which has been republished and updated (and extended in her book) since its original publication on the now defunct website decolonizingyoga.com. Barkataki suggests, and further elucidates, the following ways to "decolonize your yoga practice": "Inquire within"; "explore, learn and cite correct cultural references"; "ask ourselves and other yoga teachers, the hard questions"; "Live, know, share and practice all eight limbs of yoga, not just asana"; "be humble and honor your own and other people's journey" ("How to"). The fruits of these labors certainly ripple out to others and, perhaps, help to create bottom-up change and "our own ahimsa, or nonviolent revolution of the mind, body, and spirit" as we "decolonize ourselves [and] the yoga-industrial complex" ("How to"). I like Stanley's version of this advice: "Learn the history. Read the books. Don't pretend to be something you're not. Respect the history of Sanskrit. Respect South Asian culture. Respect what you don't know and respect your elders. Respect that the way you practice yoga has the potential of offending other people. Don't waste your time on self-flagellation—learn from your mistakes and move forward" (109). Decolonization on the individual level is a more accessible realm of change, especially since the yoga-industrial complex intersects with all of the other industrial complexes that shape our lives, our institutions, and our culture-at-large.

Barkataki's Western focus is larger than an American (U.S.) context and more easily drawn upon superficial lines of race even as she notes that "yoga means liberation from every construct, including that of race, gender, time, space, location, identity and even history herself" ("How to"). I make these critiques of social justice approaches to yoga via observations about Barkataki's work, in part, because she is an industry leader in the movement to decolonize yoga and, as her book title encapsulates, "embrace yoga's roots." Her work is valuable. Her arguments echo throughout the yoga world, in the spaces, and by the people, who Barkataki is primarily addressing— the dominant culture, the yoga-industrial complex, the superficial renderings and practices that focus on the physical practice. Ultimately, Barkataki argues for—and models—inclusivity, accessibility, intersectionality, and equity as well as embodied leadership—the path is collective and connected: "We are here together. To grow. To learn. To do better. To embrace yoga. / By listening and applying this framework to your own actions and practice, you will go far toward embracing yoga" (206). We go further together as we embrace (and critique) yoga in all its complexity and diversity, including the ways in which yoga as it has been adapted and adopted in the U.S.

*

In *Skill in Action*, Michelle Cassandra Johnson approaches the subject matter of yoga and diversity from a different angle—as "the only black girl in our [college] fitness class practicing yoga" (xii) to a social worker who "knew that [she] wanted to merge body awareness and healing with psychotherapy and social justice work" (xiii) to becoming a yogi because of her "longing for liberation in [her] body" (xiii). She explains how her "understanding of how social change occurs led [her] to merge social justice and yoga" (xiii). Johnson's book, and her arguments about yoga and social justice, are very much rooted in her personal experiences of being Black in America and in her body, and living as a survivor of sexual assault and an early diagnosis of asthma. All of these dimensions root Johnson's book more firmly in an *American* context, as opposed to Barkataki's *Western* focus. Johnson's focus on the connections between the larger culture and the culture of yoga allows her to address problems of privilege and white supremacy while also recognizing that "much of what we see in yoga practice spaces reflects these larger cultural norms" (51). A part of these cultural norms is a centering of whiteness: "Because whiteness is often unnamed, it's [sic] power to permeate a structure, institution and culture is immense" (53). Because Johnson is able to point to the larger structure, she takes the blame off of the individual white person without allowing white people to escape responsibility.

Johnson recognizes the importance of the practices she offers as extending "beyond the individual to offer resources and tools to shift institutional policies and procedures in a culture that has left all of us negatively impacted by white supremacy" (3). Toward these ends, she defines shared language—oppression, privilege, white supremacy, racism, suffering, and liberation right up front—followed by a section on approach and assumptions from "many social justice warriors [who] have put their energy into creating these assumptions" (6). Johnson weaves yoga's wisdom and potential together with her own experiences and with well-established traditions of ongoing social justice movements of all kinds in the U.S. She speaks to her own complicity in these systems alongside her commitment to "the process and the learning" (46) and she invites her readers into this process where "discomfort is the key to transformation" (46) and there is "space to fully be ourselves" (54).

*

Barkataki and Johnson both draw from their experience and racial/ethnic identity and position in relationship to global hierarchies of whiteness. No matter how carefully each of these authors navigate around the problems of whiteness, white privilege, and white supremacy, some white readers will feel personally attacked. For instance, while I find Johnson's approach to be much more focused on systems and structures and not at all an attack on white people, one of my white male nursing students took every opportunity to say how much he hated this book, admitting in his final reflection that he hated the book because he constantly felt like he was being told that "it" was his fault because he was a white male. He was the only student (so far) to have this strong reaction to the book, and I am quite certain it was because he had never been asked to think about or discuss issues of white privilege and white supremacy in his other classes (which is a travesty that speaks to the problem at hand!). Further, and like many white American males, the recent cultural turn toward a focus on diversity, equity, and inclusion and social justice had him already off balance as he met this material in an unexpected space—a nursing class about integrative healing yoga. Other readers will be tempted to think they are exempt, but both authors address that there can be no "spiritual bypassing" (Johnson 30–34) and no "permission slip to say that you are done doing the work" (Barkataki 18). Both authors encourage their readers to keep doing this hard work and whether they state it outright or not, white women (or maybe Americans, more generally) have a long road to get beyond "positionality" to critical consciousness.

Changing ourselves and our culture to be more inclusive and critically conscious is not just the work of white women, and not just the work of white people. The concept of critical consciousness (and other incarnations of radical consciousness) is a concept at least several decades old, well-worn in academic spaces. It is the predecessor to "woke," which has been used to shame people who aren't on board with someone else's progressive politics and is attacked by the right out of fear, shame, anger, and misunderstandings. In an interview in *Talking About a Revolution*, bell hooks argues that:

> ...theoretically, if white people are progressive—have truly engaged in radical consciousness or *concientización*— ... we could have a setting where everything's run by white people, but the perspectives are not biased. ... while diversity is meaningful, the essence of divesting of all of these things is that you should not need the presence of women or the presence of people of color of both genders in order to have progressive, non-biased action take place [51].

This is the world we are trying to build. Identity gets in the way. Ego gets in the way. Power structures and politics get in the way. We get in our own way. We have not yet arrived at this magical place where power no longer maps along lines of identity. These cultural trends are not particular to yoga, but perhaps our work in yoga can shine a light and lead the way. When we divest in power-over systems, we need to invest in new systems, new ways of being. We are already envisioning and enacting this world, in and out of yoga spaces, but there is more work to be done and more dimensions to navigate.

Spiritual Explorations

For most of the time I have had a yoga practice, the spiritual aspects of yoga have been the most difficult for me to wrap my head around. It is not just the fact that I am not a Christian (or of any religion, though I was raised Presbyterian) and that I am cynical and skeptical, generally. I bristle when the resources that I consult on my own personal journey of growth refer to connecting with "Spirit" or a "Higher Power" or a "Higher Self." No matter how much these sources claim that these can be God or your own interpretation of this Power, too many descriptions, uses, references, and functions read "God" to me. Maybe this is my own personal hang up. Maybe one day the clouds will part and I will see the light. Or, maybe I will remain content in my belief and understanding in the interconnectedness of all things in the universe, in my understanding that there are things that are too big (and too small) for me to see and impossible for me (or anyone) to know or fully understand. Perhaps my reverence of nature—my speechlessness at the foot of vast mountain ranges, ancient bristlecone pine trees or towering redwood trees, my unease at the edge of the depth and reach of the ocean, my awe at the endless distance of the stars and the nearness of the moon—are enough to count as "spirituality." I can certainly feel these things on a deeper level than I can express in words. Some would describe what I consider my very non-spiritual beliefs as spiritual, my observations as recognition of "God." Perhaps it is, ultimately, my inability to fix a definition, a meaning, a function, or a purpose to these bigger things that keeps me from understanding a general connection to something bigger than myself as "spirituality."

I am intrigued by people who are steadfast in their belief of God or a Higher Power or Spirit or whatever. Sometimes I'm a little bit jealous of the power of faith. Sometimes I am startled that the things I say about empowerment, transformation, feminism, and justice sound a lot like what my brother preaches to his Christian congregation. I get it, and I don't get it. Maybe what gives me pause is the extremity that often shapes spiritual beliefs. All formal religion feels like spiritual bypassing, a coping mechanism where we use spiritual practices to "avoid facing unresolved emotional issues, psychological wounds, and unfinished developmental tasks" (thank you Wikipedia!). A closer look at the two ends of the American yoga spectrum—the new age spirituality movement and the Christian adaptation of yoga—demonstrates just how far yoga can be stretched.

Two. Unpack

*

As I sat near the front row of a Kundalini yoga workshop with a very famous yoga personality at a Yoga Journal LIVE! conference in New York City, I did not know what to expect. I had known a few people who had spoken highly of Kundalini yoga and I wanted to learn more. More and more (thin, young, white, beautiful) bodies in designer-brand yoga pants continued to fill the room. The instructor's celebrity status brought over 150 people to her workshop. I was already uncomfortable. I was there to expand my yoga education and to try something new and different, something that was outside of my comfort zone. Seeing the people that this session attracted, hearing their anticipatory chatter, reminded me that this was not my kind of yoga space. Afterward, they flocked around her like a congregation of devoted followers just hoping to capture her attention, if only for a moment. And I could understand. She was impossibly beautiful and ethereal; she practically glowed in her beauty and her ability to fill and command a room full of women who were also almost impossibly beautiful.

The instructor encouraged us to embrace our truest, deepest selves. We did painful, repetitive breathing techniques along with some intense yoga postures that had my shoulders and neck screaming for relief. We were encouraged to embrace our feminine divine through particular hand positions and told to choose others if we were men. There may have been one or two men there. I was not combing the crowd to determine gender identification, but I did wonder how someone who was questioning, or transitioning, or considered themselves genderqueer or trans would feel at the invocation of these gendered instructions. I switched between the two options hoping to balance whatever feminine and masculine forces might be evoked by such gestures. At one point she noted that the feminine energy of a particular posture might increase fertility and then (somewhat jokingly) welcomed this energy in as she told us about how she hoped to have a baby soon. I immediately, and unconsciously, dropped the pose. My body reacted before my mind could catch up. I was definitely not looking for fertility.

And just when I was thinking that this workshop was not as out there as I had expected, she started to increase the intensity of her incantations. She was singing, chanting, calling the angels into the room. Around me, eyes were closed and voices were lifted. We were supposed to be bolstered by the presence of angels as they swept over us. I felt like the only skeptic in the room, and my guilt was further compounded by the fact that she was warning us against negative thoughts. I was sure that if whatever magic that was supposed to happen didn't emerge, it would be my negative thoughts that brought down the whole enterprise. I kept reminding myself to have an open mind. Instead of seeing angels, sci-fi fantasy images of winged ghost armies crushing their enemies filled my mind. I felt a great wave of nausea and discomfort, prompted by the ease with which all of these people around me slipped into this trance (or appeared to, at least). I can't help but wonder at the intensity that carries people into this flow of energy and if they can feel themselves (or something else) float away and if this is the appeal. I prefer center, grounded, an even keel.

While there is certainly variety among Kundalini yoga and it has benefited many people, for me, the spiritual aspect of this workshop felt superficial and the yoga felt esoteric and out of touch with the world we live in. It felt like a cult that swept up the vulnerable, the distraught, the desperate and disconnected. To each their own, but spiritual practices are empty without grounding in a sense of self and community and toward justice. The spiritual practice I encountered here just felt like bells and whistles and evangelical preaching—an opportunity to let go of self and join something bigger, perhaps. For me, it did not feel real. I stubbornly dug my roots into the earth and held on until the tide had passed.

*

My fear and resistance to this Kundalini yoga experience is probably not unlike that of some devout Christians when they encounter yoga. Some churches explicitly outlaw participation in yoga, Reiki, and other foreign practices that they consider to be the work of the devil. This fear leads to adaptations that are egregious appropriation—renaming poses and shifting contextualization and meaning-making. (Search the internet for, Praise Moves, for instance, and make up your own mind.) Not only is yoga not a religion, the philosophies of yoga speak to the "golden rules" of all religions. The roots of yoga are obscured and whitewashed when we attribute Bible verses or biblical names or images to "traditional" yoga poses in order to try to placate Christians. Further, using yoga as a new way to practice Christianity is insulting and arrogant; it is ignorant and unapologetic appropriation. Even so, students have shared with me some videos of pretty amazing teachers who weave yoga practice with their Christian spirituality in ways that probably feel natural and authentic to them and their followers. So, who am I to judge? Is my use of quotes from Black feminist texts exactly the same kind of mismatch? While I am all for fluidity and re-definition, sometimes cultural appropriation leads us to shut ourselves off from difference or ambiguity. Yoga leaves room for interpretation, and I encourage an embrace of this ambiguity rather than an attempt to fix it in a false place. That goes for Christian religion as much as it goes for indulgent new age spirituality or capitalistic branding. While I want to believe in yoga—that the practice of breath, awareness, and movement is enough—yoga can be used toward spirituality as well as spiritual bypassing as much as any practice.

*

In my training as a JourneyDance guide and facilitator, we explored spirituality as a connection to nature and to our inner wisdom. I had some powerful experiences during my training that are difficult to put into words, which is probably part of the point about spirituality! Through this training and my voracious reading in the field of embodied social justice, I have come to a different understanding of spirituality that clicked in a way I have not previously encountered. I became more open to what the *spiritual* can be.

In Staci K. Haines's brilliant book *The Politics of Trauma*, she details a somatic approach to trauma and healing. She describes nature as a "central resilience factor" that gives people a "connection to something more vast, felt yet unknown" (33). This bigger connection is something that I have experienced at times, as described earlier. She further explains Spirit as the "larger forces of energy, the vastness of the cosmos and unknown, and the harmonizing forces of nature" (33) and "the vast unknown, the ever-expanding universe, the energies, beyond human, that we are living within" (22). While I had thought about Spirit as a manifestation of nature, Haines's description resonates in new ways. Further, she connects this idea of Spirit to embodied transformation: "ways of being, acting, and relating [that] are aligned with what [we] most care about" (35). She writes a lot about purpose being connected to spirituality and through working with her book I was able to flesh out my purpose as: education, embodiment, and empowerment. This focus brought me closer to an understanding of all this "higher power" stuff.

Coupling this with Gail Parker's description of what a higher power is—"an ideal that lifts you beyond your everyday struggles and helps you clarify, reflect upon, and understand life from a deeper perspective, and to live it more artfully" (*Restorative* 163)—really helped these new ideas sink in. So many of us struggle to find those deeper meanings and I certainly never found them through church or the Bible (or yoga as scripture) like so many of us do. But the idea of living artfully was an idea that I could hold onto. She continues, "It is by connecting to this higher state of consciousness that you begin to reconnect to values that express your internal truth, allowing you to create meaning for yourself and make sense of things" (163). Understanding our life's path as an aspect of our spirituality shifts our entire understanding of spirituality. Our life's path is not something we are supposed to do, but it is something we have to do. It is something that we are at our core (and perhaps Christians would say it is God-given). I have often wondered where my drive and passion come from, what Octavia Butler called "positive obsession" and what my mother has referred to as "ambition." (When she saw the face I made in response, she said: "I don't mean that in a negative way!") Yoga reminds me to slow down, to let go, to find balance, and to be more than the sum of my parts.

As Parker describes the various dimensions that all come together to make us our whole selves—all of the dimensions in which we need to care for our whole selves—she further explains, "The spiritual dimension refers to our relationship to the beliefs, ideals, values, and principles that we live by; this dimension determines how we operate on the other dimensions [physical, mental/emotional, social] and how we make sense of the world" (*Transforming* 24). This description feels akin to the approach that has always resonated with me in academia—interdisciplinary critical consciousness—and in fitness/dance/yoga—cross-training and mind/body approaches. All of these allow us to be complicated, whole, multidimensional beings with enough space to inhabit contradiction. Since yoga is a life-long practice, so is our spiritual journey and that's a life worth living authentically. Life puts all kinds of hurdles in our path, but the connection to a spiritual path—to something bigger—is a ballast and a touchstone. Yoga fosters our spiritual explorations in embodied ways.

Yoga as Remedy for Addiction (and Trauma)

Spirituality is, perhaps, the only viable treatment we have found for addiction—and yoga is a powerful spiritual tool. It is also a physical, mental, and emotional tool with complementary and combined power to break through what binds us and keeps us small. Yoga is an embodied spirituality. As an integrated mind/body/spirit practice, we might argue that it works in ways that other spiritual practices cannot. Perhaps yoga alone cannot break patterns of addiction and the impacts of trauma, but yoga plus community is a powerful formula that too few people and programs utilize in the struggle against the individual and institutional impacts of addiction.

Addiction is often presented as a relatively simple matter—the story of an alcoholic's struggles until he finds himself in a Twelve-step program; the story of the alcoholic who abuses himself as much as he abuses others; the story of the alcoholic who drinks himself to a lonely or dramatic or violent death. This rendition is our most conventional American story about alcoholics, personified by Denzel Washington in *Flight* or Nicholas Cage in *Leaving Las Vegas*. I have used "he" here because, like so many of our popular narratives, most of these stories are about men. They let down their families; they let down themselves. Their wife suffers; their children suffer. They find themselves alone and self-destruct. These stories about alcoholism that dominate our patriarchal culture are not untrue, but—again, like all of our popular narratives—they are also only part of the story. The twelve-step programs of Alcoholics Anonymous (and its many incarnations) grew directly from this narrative. The remedy of AA works, but perhaps only as often as it does not work. It is almost the only game in town.

While much trial and error has been explored trying to find workable solutions for a variety of addictions, one thing remains key: addiction is a result of disconnection from others, but perhaps at least as much as from the self. The famous "rat park" study done by Dr. Bruce Alexander in the 1970s illustrates that addiction is not about the substance itself, it is about the social community. In short, when a rat was isolated and offered two water bottles, one with water and one with drugs, the isolated rat would imbibe the drug until it overdosed. When a rat was offered a "rat park" with a community of rats and activities to engage in, the rats would sometimes opt for the water bottle with the drugs, but only intermittently and they would never overdose. (Sederer) Drug addiction and alcohol addiction—as well as addictions to gambling, sex, food, exercise, shopping, and the electronic gadgets we are chained to (and even to buying classical music recordings, as Dr. Gabor Maté writes about his own struggles with addiction in his important book *In the Realm of Hungry Ghosts: Close Encounters with Addiction*)—is all about filling a hole, feeding an emptiness, whether we are conscious of this gaping hole and ravenous hunger or not. These addictions are also most often attached to unresolved trauma.

Addiction is as simple as this, but also far more complicated; and clearly we have yet to figure out how to address the problems of addiction in our society. The twelve-step programs of AA and its progeny are, to date, the best thing we've got. (Perhaps because they provide community connections.) Mostly, we have yet to figure out how to address the social and cultural (and economic) problems that create an environment in which addiction exists and most recovery programs treat mind and spirit but not so much the body. The "rat park" that we humans live in becomes more and more devoid of social connections, embodied practices, and deeper meanings. We could blame technology for this disconnection, but it is only one of the factors. The healthcare system treats symptoms rather than the underlying problems—of any and all illnesses and diseases—and prescribes a magical pill for whatever ails us, physical or mental. The implications of this ideology reverberate across differences of class, race, and gender with frightening consequences. The rich get richer and the poor get poorer. And we blame individuals for the problems that originate in cultural patterns and belief systems.

*

When I took a yoga training for addiction and recovery, I began to understand addiction in a radically different dimension. I could also see very clearly how my issues with codependency and work (and, at times, food and alcohol and marijuana and sex) were coping mechanisms teetering on the edge of addictions. They were substitutions for a deeper connection with myself and, perhaps, a deeper connection with that Higher Power that I could not force myself to believe in. I stopped thinking about addiction as a problem that other people struggled with and started thinking of it as a problem that I also struggle with—and that maybe all of us struggle with in some way. I was able to see more dimensions of addiction intellectually, but I was also going through a difficult period in my life, on my journey to find myself and manage my PTSD, and there are always more lessons to learn.

Halfway through the training (which was online), I felt like I was going to completely unravel. My head was spinning and I could not find my center. I was trying all of my tools, desperately. And then something from the training hit me: HALT. Hungry, angry, lonely, tired. Recognizing my HALT symptoms and breathing helped me to stop the spinning, shift back to center, and forgive myself for losing control. This is a longer story, but the point is that we all have tendencies toward addiction and we all need connections to tools and people. We all use substances or behavior or negative (or positive!) thinking patterns to avoid the things in our lives that are tough to face. The more we can recognize these tendencies in ourselves, the more we can tap into tools like yoga and embodied movements to help us keep our balance and make connections within and beyond ourselves.

Yoga has been used to treat not only the individual in recovery, but also to create a community for those in need of recovery.

Nikki Myers launched Yoga of Twelve-Step Recovery (Y12SR) in 2004. Y12SR combines a "group sharing circle, and an intentional yoga class," trains and certifies instructors in this approach to recovery, and maintains a database of donation-based classes online and across the U.S. Books like Tommy Rosen's *Recovery 2.0* speak to the power of both the Twelve Steps and yoga (specifically Kundalini yoga and, generally, meditation). Rosen's journey is offered up in his book as inspiration to others who are searching for a remedy. It is both a wide and narrow net, offering yoga as a supplement or complement to the Twelve Steps, examining many aspects of his life in great depth while leaving his social and cultural power, and class and gender privilege, largely unchecked and offering a very specific kind of yoga practice as example. We need resources like Rosen's book and Y12SR, but we also need to unpack other aspects of our experience and larger cultural incubator.

Because addiction is a rampant problems across all sectors of our society and culture (and our world), it does not make sense to locate the problems of addiction in the realm of the individual. Jacoby Ballard brings an important dimension to this conversation, writing about addiction (and trauma, and so much more) in relation to yoga and the queer community, most importantly connecting back to larger systems and structures. They write, "the source of our trauma is ultimately injustice, oppression, colonization, and capitalism. Addiction is the result of the trauma of injustice" (167). Emotional balance, breath, consciousness (or awareness), interoception, imagination, and connection with and beyond the self are powerful yoga tools that remedy addiction and reverberate beyond the individual. The healing offered through yoga—for addiction and trauma and for a whole host of physical/mental/emotion ailments—is multidimensional, integrative, holistic, and embodied. We have only begun to tap into this power individually, let alone collectively.

Trauma: From the Individual to the Collective

When I first began to study trauma, it was largely in an effort to work toward healing my own trauma. For years, yoga (and fitness) had been a semi-conscious stop-gap measure—it helped me to stay afloat, but I was not yet ready to heal. When I began to learn about trauma in relation to the tools that yoga provides, I quickly learned that I was already teaching trauma-informed yoga, in part because of my training, which emphasized teaching to "every body," and in part because my academic training and teaching are so closely tied to social justice. Jacoby Ballard also writes about their experience in the two spheres of social justice work and healing work, noting that he has seen more people doing social justice work engaging in healing work and more people engaging in healing work engaging in social justice work (194). Angela Davis makes a similar argument: "I think our notions of what counts as radical have changed over time. Self-care and healing and attention to the body and the spiritual dimension—all of this is now a part of radical social justice struggles. That wasn't the case before" (qtd. in Hobart and Kneese). We can't make all yoga spaces "safe," but we can make all yoga spaces more critically conscious, more inviting, less hierarchical, and more open as "brave spaces," as inclusive spaces of community healing. Many of us make similar arguments, including Heyman, Ballard, and Raffo (104) (and see Arao and Clemens). The shift from the use of "safe" to "brave" and away from the use of the word "trigger" toward "activate" (or other less-charged words) to describe nervous system responses is an important shift in activist and yoga spaces.

Because injustice and oppression are key causes of trauma, and because trauma leads not only to addiction, but to a variety of other social and cultural issues as well as physical, mental, and emotional problems that impact individuals, families, communities and beyond, people and organizations have sought many different remedies to the impacts of trauma. However, it is becoming more and more apparent that we can really only treat trauma with an embodied approach. As Jacoby Ballad argues, "If we are only addressing the source of our trauma through activism, artistic expression, or education, but not healing our bodies, hearts, and minds, then we inevitably recreate trauma in our lives" (168). Jacoby Ballard's chapter, "Injustice Produces Trauma; Healing Creates Conditions for Justice" in *A Queer Dharma* is absolutely brilliant and an important addition to our collective conversation about trauma. Go read it now. I will wait.

In and out of yoga spaces we may not recognize what we are experiencing as a *trauma* response. Trauma can be unconscious, undiscovered, unresolved. Trauma is complex—and then there's complex trauma, collective trauma, childhood trauma, historical trauma, intergenerational trauma and more categories that speak to the many insidious manifestations of trauma. As Susan Raffo (and others) argue, "There is no such thing as individual trauma, even though we sometimes experience it individually. Each moment of absence, of disconnection, swirls around and between many different lives and generations" (223). And we may never *resolve* trauma. But what is abundantly clear is that trauma lives in the body. And if trauma is not addressed through embodied movements, it will remain and fester. Toward embodied approaches to trauma, social justice work and healing work are becoming more closely aligned.

*

Social justice approaches to yoga that highlight trauma build upon works that explore and elucidate the impacts, manifestations, and insidious workings of trauma in a variety of contexts. A seminal work is Bessel van der Kolk's book *The Body Keeps the Score: Brain, Mind, and Body in the Healing of Trauma*, published in 2015 after three decades of working with trauma survivors. This big, heavy book is not a light read, but it is a vitally important one. While he describes a number of innovative treatments, including neurofeedback, sports, and drama, it is no surprise that meditation and yoga are two treatments that have gained more and more traction. The impacts of childhood trauma are one of the most fascinating and important topics that van der Kolk writes about, and this work has been taken up by doctors and mental health professionals as well as yoga teachers and trainers and somatic practitioners.

In *Therapeutic Yoga for Trauma Recovery*, in addition to the big ideas made accessible—like polyvagal theory and embodiment and the easy-to-follow and accessible "Journey of Practices"—Arielle Schwartz makes parallels between the steps of trauma recovery and yoga practice. Both "tend to be more circuitous than linear" (2). Schwartz leads the reader through a healing journey that starts with "Create Your Sacred Space" and "Choice and Freedom" and continues with information about the eight limbs of yoga and a plethora of physical, mental, and spiritual guidance. Perhaps most important to a larger understanding of trauma and yoga, early in the Introduction she draws direct parallels between "personal suffering" as it is "compounded by the collective trauma that results from pandemics, climate change, or systemic racism" and further exacerbated by "legacy wounds of unhealed trauma from previous generations, which are passed down in the form of emotional and physical tension" (xxix). While she shares personal information in the Preface, Schwartz is a guide, and other than the pictures of her that are sprinkled throughout the book, her personal story is not the driver; her wealth of professional knowledge, insights, and experience are what helps individual readers move through this journey of healing trauma.

Staci K. Haines writes about trauma in groundbreaking clarity in her book *The Politics of Trauma: Somatics, Healing, and Social Justice*. Haines describes the way that the soma (a holistic view of mind/body/spirit) "organizes itself" (75) in relation to trauma: "We become organized for danger, abandonment, and humiliation—without a way to regain safety, belonging, and dignity holistically" (76). She further explains that we become our habits and survival strategies and that these come at a cost to our bodies as well as our families and communities (96–7). We embody our survival strategies "not only in our neuronal pathways, but also in our muscles and tissues" (77) and once embodied, these strategies become "less and less conscious to us and more 'just how things are'" (77). We start to think that we are flawed, that this is just "who I am" instead of realizing that we have been shaped by circumstances outside of our control (146–7) because trauma not only happens on the individual level, but also on the systemic level. She reminds us that we can't just talk our way out of trauma. We can't just fix it or override it; "something deeper and more transformative is called for" (123). One of the most important arguments that she makes in her book is that we can't just treat the individual as an isolated case of trauma and that we need "liberatory community and collective practices, connected to transformative systemic change" (46) in order to cultivate, embodied, lasting, transformative change.

When it comes to trauma (and so many other things!) individual healing and structural transformation are both necessary. In Nadine Burke Harris's *The Deepest Well: Healing the Long-Term Effects of Childhood Trauma and Adversity*, she traces the ways in which childhood trauma and adversity impact the stress response system and the ways in which toxic stress damages an individual's health over their lifetime as well as into the next generation. Toxic stress is a public health crisis and while she recognizes the systemic issues, her focus is on the ways in which we can treat the impacts of trauma before they manifest into more serious illnesses. She advocates for including universal screening for ACEs (Adverse Childhood Experiences) during routine pediatric check-ups and approaching medical care through multidisciplinary team approaches. She notes that adverse childhood experiences impact every sector of society (across race, class, and gender, for instance) and that we need the "*same* fundamental approach to treatment for us *all*" (195). "We are all equally susceptible and equally in need of help when adversity strikes. And that is what a lot of folks *don't* want to hear" (194). It is easier to imagine that toxic stress only impacts those most marginalized in American society, and it is easier to blame the environment or the "weakness" of individuals. But socioeconomic inequalities only exacerbate the impacts of toxic stress. In *Embodied Self Awakening: Somatic Practices for Trauma Healing and Spiritual Evolution* Nityda Gessel argues that "trauma can be that which is too much, too fast, too soon" as well as "too little for too long" (5). The former means that our nervous system is overwhelmed; the second means that "our spiritual needs are not being met" (5). This second meaning meshes with Harris's arguments and illustrates the impacts of socioeconomic disparities. While "too little for too long" certainly impacts white-bodied people, it disproportionately impacts people of color.

As Harris argues, by intervening before biological changes to the neurologic, endocrine, and immune systems can cause bigger problems, we can not only help people live happier, more healthful lives, we can also reduce the costs associated with treating some of the most common health problems in the U.S. like diabetes, asthma, heart disease, obesity, and more. She writes, "the solutions are as simple as reducing the dose of adversity and enhancing the ability of caregivers to be buffers" (211). Through sleep, exercise, nutrition, mindfulness, mental health, and healthy relationships, children and adults can curb the impacts of toxic stress. Harris's book is worth a read. Not only is it well-written, interesting, and accessible, it is revolutionary. As she argues, "I believe that when we each find the courage to look this problem in the face, we will have the power to transform not only our health, but our world" (222). People like Harris are working toward this vision every day.

One of the arguments that Harris makes (and many others, including myself!) is that we need to take care of ourselves in order to care for others. As I note above, Harris explains the importance of caregivers to be "buffers" and they cannot be buffers if they don't deal with their own stress-response systems. This is especially the case when it comes to intergenerational trauma. While intergenerational trauma comes from many different sources, ethnic and race-based trauma come with their own challenges, especially since simply living in the U.S is a constant source of trauma (re)activation. Resmaa Menakem illustrates various impacts of intergenerational trauma in a U.S. context, breaking down the impacts and remedies for white-bodied people, Black people, and for the police body. As a therapist and founder of Cultural Somatics and creator of Somatic Abolitionism, he blends theory and practice and encourages us to proactively move trauma out of our bodies so that we don't "blow" it through other bodies. Much of what Menakem offers overlaps with yoga, but Gail Parker explicitly links yoga as a means for transforming ethnic and race-based trauma.

Gail Parker's book *Restorative Yoga for Ethnic and Race-Based Stress and Trauma* and the related book, *Transforming Ethnic and Race-Based Traumatic Stress with Yoga: Rest, Reflect, and Renew*, are packed with insight and wisdom from Parker's life and practice and from yoga traditions. The latter offers practical tools that include restorative postures with simple instructions and affirmations that complement the postures. And while the content is focused around the topic of ethnic and race-based stress, the practices are universal. In fact, in *Transforming*, she begins the introduction by noting that "regardless of race and ethnicity, we are all impacted by its damaging effects, from those who are wounded to those who intentionally or unwittingly do the wounding" (19). Thus, Parker's books are important for all of us to read, and to re-read, and to engage in the practices that she provides in *Transforming*. Parker's books allow us to find common ground, but also enable us all to reckon with the impacts of racism and white supremacy, individually and collectively. In the chapter on authenticity, she notes that "trauma often leads people to become seekers as a way to come to terms with or understand themselves at deeper levels beyond culture, race, and ethnicity" (86). As Harris argues, trauma impacts all of us. Some become seekers. Some become addicts. Some both. Some hurt themselves and/or other people, on large or small scales. There is so much pain in this world; we see the impacts everywhere. The lens of trauma is one way that we can come together toward healing and transformation.

Parker continues, "Many trauma survivors are drawn to yoga practices intuitively…" (86). Yoga's draw speaks to the power of yoga to heal and transform, to buffer the stress response system, as Harris might argue. In a note at the beginning of *Transforming*, she clarifies her language, distinguishing between "transformation" and "healing," which she uses "sometimes interchangeably" (13). "Healing," she argues "is a term we use when we discuss illness or injury. Racial stress and trauma are emotional injuries that, left unhealed, become chronic and can lead to negative health outcomes" (13). This is the kind of healing that Harris's approach tackles. "Transformation, on the other hand, suggests change—in this case, positive change that leads to growth" (13). The emotional and spiritual growth that yoga provides is a foundation for transformation.

Parker's books offer a wealth of insights beyond the particular modality of restorative yoga and beyond the specific focus on ethnic and race-based trauma. Her yoga wisdom is born in an American context. In *Restorative Yoga for Ethnic and Race-Based Stress and Trauma*, Parker reminds us that:

> Reaching out and speaking your truth require stepping into your vulnerability. It is usually not a comfortable feeling and requires strength. We have to fortify ourselves internally so we are not derailed by our emotions when we get triggered by racial insults, or burn out because we are trying so hard to make a difference, or freeze in the face of racially insensitive behaviors that require a response [95].

As we have unpacked issues surrounding yoga—and embedded in American yoga—we may have been "triggered"—activated or agitated. As Parker reminds us, "This journey is not a safe one. It is a brave one. Disrupting the status quo involves risk.... Sometime we have to be willing to do it scared" (95). But being and doing while scared never give us an excuse to treat people harshly, which happens all the time in everyday struggles as well as in movements toward social justice. Fortifying ourselves takes practice, self-compassion, patience, and a host of other qualities that yoga can help us foster. "This means establishing a relationship of mutuality, reciprocity, and trust by showing up safe for one another. This is how we grow together" (95). Parker's wisdom reminds us what is at stake and that we can't keep doing things the way they have always been done. We need to expand the scope of our vision—for ourselves, our communities, and for our American legacy. Queering yoga is one such expansion.

Queering Yoga

Queer is a reclaimed word. It is an umbrella term that denotes a spectrum of identities and sexualities that have been marginalized and demonized. I like this term because it is inclusive, *political*, and ambiguous; and because the word also means unusual, not normal, odd, eccentric, and unconventional. To some people, the word queer brings up feelings associated with past injustices; to others, it is a threat to "traditional" (read: religious, conservative) American values. To queer something, as Jacoby Ballard describes, is to "critique, challenge, and transform toward something more radical—that is deeply rooted in truth, love, and justice" (117). The "viral quote" from Black Canadian poet Brandon Wint explains: "'Not queer like gay. Queer like, escaping definition. Queer like some sort of fluidity and limitlessness at once. Queer like a freedom too strange to be conquered. Queer like the fearlessness to imagine what love can look like and pursue it'" (qtd. in Taylor 116–17). Critiquing what we love is an American legacy that reaches toward truth and justice. There are many ways to be queer and many ways to practice and offer queer yoga.

Ballard writes about some of the ways that we can queer yoga and the importance of creating opportunities and spaces for queer people to do yoga together, "surrounding ourselves with people and environments that nourish us" (166). As Ballard argues, "Society is constantly telling queer and trans people that we shouldn't exist, through overt and subversive forms of oppression" (164). Because trauma lives in the body, yoga provides the opportunity for queer people "to be in their bodies as their whole selves" (165) and to practice "letting go of shame, of guilt, of shields that we may hold in our bodies, hearts, and minds" (172). This is no small thing. We all deserve to be in our bodies as our whole selves.

Ballard's work is only one example of people who are offering ideas, practices, and spaces for queer yoga, and queer yoga for youth can be particularly powerful in helping young people navigate their bodies and identities. Closer to my home in Maine, the Queer Yoga Youth Project launched in 2023, "aims to offer valuable resources for queer youth to safely connect with their bodies, develop practical skills they can use to self-regulate, and learn more about how to support their general wellness" (Sea Change). However, quite obviously, such opportunities are much easier to find in urban areas like Portland, Maine, and not so easy to find in smaller cities, towns, and rural areas—the rest of Maine. This is one of the reasons why it was important to me to offer queer yoga to my community when I opened The Spiral Goddess Collective. I wanted to bring my particular approach to yoga and movement, which is *queer*—unconventional, radical, inclusive, trauma-informed, creative, and "deeply rooted in truth, love, and justice," as Jacoby Ballard describes.

Despite my professional life as a professor and fitness instructor—both things that appear to be the realms of the extrovert—I am a shy, introverted, home body who likes to spend time by myself—usually with a book and preferably with a cat or two or three. I'm not the type to yell from rooftops or wave a flag in a parade regardless of how passionate I am. When Hannah Gadsby asks where the introverted queers are in her brilliant stand-up special, *Nanette*, I dare to whisper "right here" and feel seen. Opening the Spiral Goddess Collective was an opportunity for me to be more brave, more open, and more in line with my values. Our space and our offerings push up against the boundaries of the norms of fitness spaces as well as the norms of social justice movements. We center feminine qualities and values like collaboration, compassion, empathy, nurturing, and flow. The Spiral Goddess is not just a symbol for women—it is an archetype that informs what we birth into the world, how we use our energy, how we treat ourselves and each other, and how we connect our inner and outer worlds. The Spiral Goddess symbol and feminine values push back against a world where individuals are forced to choose one side of the gender binary, which can lead to violence against ourselves and others. And this is where queer yoga enters the picture.

*

It is fairly easy to see the problems with mainstream American spaces that marginalize and demonize queer ideas and queer bodies. But what, exactly, is "queer yoga"? Jacoby Ballard describes queer yoga as having the following qualities: Not using gendered language, including queer realities and contexts, queering gear, bringing on the "sass," recognizing the political aspect of a queer identity, using queer music (validating queer experience), and teaching trauma-informed (170–5). The umbrella of queer holds a spectrum of difference; thus, queer yoga must as well. In my queer yoga workshop, this is how I present additional qualities of queer yoga: to bring conscious, critical, intersectional reflection to the practice(s) of yoga; to expand the spectrum of possibility beyond the male/female binary; to offer inclusive, accessible yoga and for LGBTQIA+ affinity groups when possible; to give back to the community through collective care initiatives; to create a trauma-informed container for brave exploration of body/mind/spirit as well as connections to each other and with everything bigger than we are; and to provide opportunities to experience an authentic, embodied practice that meets each body and each mind/body where they are.

Because I am a different queer body/mind/spirit, and because I meet queerness and queer community in different ways than Ballard, it only makes sense that I would offer a different version of queer yoga. Queer is a big umbrella and, thus, so is Queer Yoga. Jacoby Ballard writes about the importance of shared cultural references and using music by queer-identified artists and queer cultural icons. Music is powerful—the sounds and vibrations, the beat, the cultural resonance, and the lyrical messaging. In most yoga classes I choose music that is relaxing and healing (literally, solfeggio frequencies for healing). But when I teach "queer yoga," I mix in songs that are from *my* queer experience as music moves out of the background and becomes a part of our celebratory, communal practice. Thus, my queer music is more from the femme side of the queer spectrum, which also obviously resonates with the theme of The Spiral Goddess Collective: "Chasing Rainbows" by Big Freedia, featuring Kesha; "Crimson and Clover" by Joan Jett & The Blackhearts; "Superpower" by Adam Lambert; "Yoga" by Janelle Monáe, featuring Jindeena; "Can't Help but Fly" by Climbing Poetree, featuring be steadwell; "As Is" by Ani DiFranco; "Float" by Janelle Monáe, Seun Kuti, and Egypt 80; and "Breathe In" by be steadwell. These songs inspire my practice and the queer practice of yoga that I attempt to offer with authenticity and humility instead of shame and doubt.

As more yoga teachers claim their own particular queer identities, the scope of queer yoga broadens and shines its rainbow into all kinds of mainstream spaces. And as more mainstream, white, middle-class spaces become inclusive of all kinds of difference, the radical potential of yoga disrupts yoga business as usual and transforms itself and the world around it. We are only beginning to witness the ripples of this version of American yoga. Transformative healing happens from the inside out and the outside in. When we move our minds/bodies together, we are stronger—we are a collective of power and potential!

Ability and Disability in American Yoga Spaces

Because American yoga is so focused on the physical practice of yoga, it follows that yoga often leaves out those bodies and minds that don't fit in inaccessible spaces. American yoga has not even begun to address its inherent ableism. Jivana Heyman writes that "the way we have equated advanced yoga practice with physical ability is a form of deeply ingrained ableism" (107). He describes ableism as "the incorrect notion that some bodies are better than other bodies, as well as the idea that disabled bodies need to be fixed or healed" (107). Disability is often seen as something to fear from those of us who enjoy the privilege of an able body. As Heyman notes, "we are trained from a young age that disability, illness, old age, fatness, and any other differences from some supposed norm are to be avoided and shamed" (107–8). However, disability is more of a norm than American culture and society is willing to admit. Part of the reason that mainstream society and culture fail to understand and accommodate disability is because of the fear that we have surrounding disability. On some level we might know, and even understand, that an able body can become a disabled body at any moment due to any variety of circumstances outside of our control. The physical and mental deteriorate with and age as well as mis-use and dis-use. We might think that we can medicate away mental disabilities. We often blame people for their disabilities—whether they were born disabled or became disabled. We think that we will never end up like *them*, but aging and accidents (and violence and trauma) bring disability that we can't always avoid, manage, or buy our way out of.

I will admit that for most of my life and career I thought very little about disability. As an able-bodied person, I did not have to think about it—and this is the most basic definition of privilege. I would even sometimes get disgruntled by the idea of having to think about ability as an aspect of intersectionality. But this was another kind of fear—a fear of the unknown. I didn't know very much about disability, and I had the privilege to avoid it, and so I did. But I would feel uneasy about glossing over something I knew I didn't understand. This changed when my university selected "Disability Visibility" (and the book of essays by the same title, edited by Alice Wong) for our 2022–23 academic theme and I began to educate myself. And suddenly I realized what an ignorant and ableist jerk I had been! I also realized that I was not, perhaps, as able-bodied as I thought I was. We all need this wake up call.

*

Leah Lakshmi Piepzna-Samarasinha's book, *Care Work: Dreaming Disability Justice*, is pivotal for an understanding of disability in the context of care work, a category that contextualizes yoga and the dis/ability aspects of this practice in important ways. When we understand yoga as care work, we find that caring for oneself and caring for others are intertwined. We also understand that care work often falls on the shoulders of women and people of color in private and public care scenarios. Yoga can be care work that liberates and transforms the individual in the form of self-care and ripples outward to liberate and transform members of our communities, but only if we make yoga more accessible to everyone—to every mind and body—not just in pithy catch phrases, but in actual practices. Jivana Heyman founded the Accessible Yoga Association, "an international nonprofit organization dedicated to increasing access to the yoga teachings." His calling, and his career, have been in service to the idea of making yoga accessible and his version of accessibility goes beyond the physical practice of yoga. He writes, "Ironically, asana is what makes yoga accessible and often inaccessible simultaneously" (174). Indeed. In *Yoga Revolution*, Heyman offers many accessible yoga tools and approaches to yoga (visualization, meditation, and bed yoga, to name a few) and one of his chapters in the third section "Yoga in Practice" emphasizes "Caring for Yourself with Yoga." Many other yoga teachers offer these tools and practices in conjunction with the physical practice of yoga.

Heyman is not the first or only person or organization to call for yoga that meets "every body" where they are. For instance, Jessamyn Stanley's book is titled *Every Body Yoga*, Dianne Bondy's book is *Yoga for Everyone*, and the yoga teacher training program that I am trained in also includes yoga for "every body" in its mission. For years, the Facebook group I created to complement my free community offerings used the phrase "Yoga for Every Mind/Body" (it still does) even though I don't use this phrase to describe or title my classes. Even as we proclaim this more universal quality of yoga—which is absolutely true only because yoga is so many things and one or more aspects of yoga will always be accessible to everyone regardless of the body they are in—it is rare to find a singular yoga class, or a singular yoga book, that is able to provide yoga for *every* body. We are simply too diverse. Yoga for every body is a wonderfully inclusive slogan and marketing tool, but if we make this claim and a body is left out, then we may be inadvertently causing harm. We may be less inclusive than we intend to be.

Making yoga spaces more accessible is not always easy. When I opened The Spiral Goddess Collective, the space that was the impetus to create my "business" and community center just happened to be a space on the 4th floor of an inaccessible historic building. This location limits my ability to bring yoga to those who cannot climb four flights of stairs. However, I try to counter this limitation by offering yoga via Zoom once a week and by taking yoga and movement practices into other community spaces. This is a small, but not insignificant, act that attempts to make what is inaccessible because of physical location more accessible. There is more that we can do, but we are also limited by access to resources and the limitations of space and time.

Trauma-informed yoga begins to make yoga more accessible to people who are neurodivergent, and by offering choice, also makes strides toward making yoga accessible to different kinds of bodies. Chair yoga offers options to those who need to be seated, but is often seen as a practice for only those who need to remain seated (which is usually associated with the elderly) and not as a form of yoga that any body can benefit from. The more we move away from understanding yoga as a physical practice, the more we are able to bring accessible yoga to people who are disabled physically and mentally. And the more we recognize how we can all benefit from the philosophical and meditative aspects of yoga practice. Movement can be glacial, incremental, and profound.

Ultimately, as the 2022 book title from Leah Lakshmi Piepzna-Samarasinha proclaims, *The Future Is Disabled*. Our collective future is disabled. As we age, we become disabled. As toxic chemicals inundate our food and water supplies, we become disabled. As medical care becomes more expensive and more difficult to access, we become disabled. And the prospect of this disabled future, as she contextualizes it, is not something to mourn, but something to celebrate. As she writes, "at the core of my work and life is the belief that disabled wisdom is the key to our survival and expansion. Crip genius is what will keep us all alive and bring us home to the just and survivable future we all need. If we have a chance in hell of getting there" (18). We need to listen to Crip genius. We need to embrace disability as a new norm and follow the lead of the queer and trans BIPOC leaders of the Disability Justice movement. We need to prioritize a version of universal design—in and out of yoga spaces.

*

I close this section about disability—and the "Unpack" chapter—with the example of yoga nidra as a powerful tool for individual and collective transformation. This deep rest form of yoga takes us into a meditative state where we can access layers of ourselves in different ways and integrate the unconscious aspects of our experience in this world. Deep rest has been found to have a number of benefits that span the physical, mental, emotional, and neurological—from physical healing to better learning to neuroplasticity to a method to increase productivity. Neuroscientist, Andrew Huberman, coined the term "non-sleep deep rest" (NSDR) to describe this method of deep relaxation and he has a ton of information available via his free Huberman Lab podcast and online resources. Scientists are very good at discovering what yogis have known for centuries and making it more mainstream.

Yoga nidra is sometimes referred to as "yogic sleep" and is not a form of yoga that most Americans would recognize, let alone opt for in their pursuit of yoga. I have really only begun to explore this form of yoga, which is far deeper and richer than I can begin to express here. Yoga nidra includes a body scan, which can be performed on any kind of body, able or not. It improves body awareness and we can also explore the power of connection to ourselves and the alignment of our heart's desire and higher purpose. We can go deeper and tap into our nervous system's healing functions. Thus, the mind/body/spirit practice of yoga nidra is an accessible, integrated, and transformative practice that might be spread more widely by the American yoga powers that be—because Americans need more rest, more connection, and more introspection, even if we don't know we do. I return to yoga as rest in the "Imagine" section—we can imagine rest as a crucial part of our practice on and off the mat.

Interlude:
Yoga Tools Off the Mat

In the fast-paced, exercise-oriented world of American Yoga there are many reasons why a focus on the physical postures of yoga—the official poses, the classic *asanas*—are seen as the most important part of yoga. They are often the most accessible to us, especially when we are first exploring what yoga is (and they feel good!). We might struggle with the desire (or obsession) to do the poses in the right way. But, like so much of life, there is not only one right way. Further, just because something is right for one person doesn't mean that it is right for another person. Just because I find joy, stillness, and enlightenment in a particular pose doesn't mean that everyone will too. We should do the yoga postures that we like, but maybe we should also do the ones that we don't like as much. Always, we should modify to feel comfortable in a pose. We can discover where a physical pose—especially those we don't like so much—might take us mentally, emotionally, spiritually. Better yet, we might delve deeper than the physical aspects of a pose and maybe even stop being attached to the idea of poses in the first place. Poses/postures/*asanas* are just *shapes* that we make. The shapes are a gateway.

This interlude considers a variety of ideas and tools that are off the mat—some of which aren't really yoga at all. We start with one of the most difficult aspects of yoga for busy, productivity-driven Americans—slowing down.

Slowing Down (the Mind and the Body)

The busy, spinning mind that so many of us experience is often referred to as the monkey mind, and has been noted in ancient times as well as modern. Yoga can help us to be in the now, the present moment. It can help us to focus on our breath, to be still. By matching our breath to our movement, we can let both slow down. Yoga can help us to step away from the frenetic pace of our lives and to focus our attention on the body—what the body needs, where it is in space, what we want to do with it, where we want to take it, and how we are feeling. In American culture, slowing down is frowned upon. Slow is weak. Slow is lazy. Old people are slow. Disabled people are slow. Slow gets in the way. We don't have time for slow! But slow is powerful. Slow might be something we have to seek, something we have to make room for—a way to be purposeful and powerful in our lives and in our movements. Slowing down is one way of taking care of ourselves.

Self-Care, Self-Compassion, and Radical Self-Love

I first heard the term self-care many years ago at a National Women's Studies Association conference, at a panel with the Crunk Feminist Collective. Brittany Cooper spoke to the importance of self-care, following the well-worn quote (which is a prolific meme) by Audre Lorde: "Caring for myself is not self-indulgence, it is self-preservation, and that is an act of political warfare," which she wrote in a 1988 essay collection, *A Burst of Light*. The concept blew my mind! Was I allowed to practice self-care? Like many ideas foundational to social justice and women's empowerment, the concept has its roots in Black feminist movement. It took me many more years to give myself permission to practice self-care and it is still something I have to constantly give myself permission to do, even though I give my students permission all the time by making self-care a mandatory assignment.

The first requirement of self-care is that we earn the right to claim self-care through service to others. It is not just about having "girl time" or a time out. Self-care is not about pedicures and mimosas (though these things might be involved). It is about recharging our resources so that we have enough energy to sustain us and more energy to give without giving too much of ourselves. The well-worn idea that "you can't pour from an empty cup" is helpful for understanding the toll that giving and giving and giving can take on a person. The other analogy of putting on your oxygen mask first is a popular way of considering self-care and illustrates the deep divide between privilege and oppression in understandings and discussions of self-care. If someone has never flown on an airplane, this analogy will not resonate. Many women and femmes are tasked with taking care of everyone first; we often put this expectation on ourselves. Kids, spouses, family, friends, and our culture all demand it of us. And many non-white women, past and present, have sacrificed the care of their families to care for the families of white women because this sacrifice is what white supremacy demands for survival.

At its root, self-care is about being in touch with ourselves enough to determine what we need to sustain ourselves and nurture ourselves to grow. We have to do this work to care for ourselves because our institutions do not prioritize our health and well-being. Bo Forbes talks about self-care in relationship to restorative yoga and asks what it might mean to literally give ourselves the support and comfort that we need. Many of us do not even consider that giving ourselves support is something that we are allowed to do. In her book, *Set Boundaries, Find Peace: A Guide to Reclaiming Yourself*, Nedra Glover Tawwab writes: "The root of self-care is setting boundaries: it's saying no to something in order to say yes to your own emotional, physical, and mental well-being" (6). Setting boundaries might be the most important self-care practice. For some people, boundaries are easy. I'm always in awe of these individuals. For others, myself included, boundaries are a constant struggle. I'm still working on identifying the need for boundaries, figuring out what a boundary might look like, establishing that boundary, and holding it.

Along these lines, self-care might not be something that we do; it might be about doing less. It might be about giving ourselves permission to relax, to produce less, to take time off and enjoy life. I assign a self-care project in almost every academic class I teach and

I find that students often have a whole list of things they are going to do for self-care. I suggest that these students scrap that list and do nothing as their self-care project. Sometimes I beg students to do nothing or to see the value in doing less. Many students cannot sustain self-care throughout a semester, even if it is just a little thing or doing nothing. This assignment ends with a reflection, so even when the self-care fails, the lessons that students take from the project are what is important. And in this reflection, most students find success. Some even find new ways of living.

Self-compassion is a kind of self-care and has to do with countering and re-scripting negative self-talk and treating ourselves with the same compassion that we show other people in our life. (Kristin Neff has a ton of resources and research on the topic of self-compassion.) If we cannot be compassionate toward ourselves, then how can we be compassionate toward other people? When I started studying self-care, self-compassion, and radical self-love, I started to notice just how toxic we are to ourselves. On a trip to Chicago for my mother's 70th birthday, I was appalled at the way that my sister talked about other people, constantly criticizing. And then I realized that she was just as critical of herself, if not more so. This dual internal/external dynamic of criticism is not unusual. Several months later I visited my mother-in-law and could not believe how negative she was toward herself. She beat herself up about the smallest things, calling herself stupid when she got lost going to a place she had never been before, punishing herself for making small mistakes, refusing to go in the pool at her retirement complex (when no one else was there!) because she was too fat and did not want to be seen. She had been doing this to herself for her entire life and it devastated me to think that at nearly 80 years old she could not let go of some of her self-criticism. Seeing these behaviors in my family members, very quickly helped me shed most of my self-deprecating thoughts and behaviors. Few of these women are ready to hear that it is okay to love themselves despite whatever flaws they imagine. This self-criticism is a cultural norm. Witnessing it is devastating.

Making a commitment to self-care can also be about practicing self-love and self-compassion. For a long time I didn't think twice about the concept of self-love. I took it as a given that I loved myself.

But one day (with the help of mental health therapy), I realized that I had no love for myself, and that the way I treated myself and gave all of myself to others was detrimental to my health and well-being as well as my relationships. It was a long hard road to self-love and one day it just clicked and I knew I had never felt that kind of love before. Still, I need reminders, reconnections. Sonya Renee Taylor's movement, website, and book, *The Body Is Not an Apology*, revolutionize the idea of self-love—radical self-love—the best kind of self and community care. My students love this book and most devoured it in a couple of days, even though I had stretched the assigned reading out over several weeks of my Embodied Social Justice course. As she explains, "using the term radical elevates the reality that our society requires a drastic political, economic, and social reformation in the ways in which we deal with bodies and body difference" (8). She connects self-love to the larger systems and structures that we intervene in when we learn to have love for ourselves. For instance, she argues, "When we decide that people's bodies are wrong because we don't understand them, we are trying to avoid the discomfort of divesting from an entire body-shame system" (21). I could quote almost every sentence in this golden book. Taylor writes accessibly and she only asks of her reader what she is willing to ask of herself. Her message is inspiring: "…we must become architects of a world that works for everybody and every body" (82). Ultimately, self-care is not so much about the individual, despite the prominent centering of the self; self-care is a means toward collective care and transformation of dominant ideologies.

Alongside commercial and corporate narratives that position self-care as a kind of personal responsibility, self-care is becoming increasingly recognized as an important practice especially for those most oppressed by systems and structures and for activists working to change these systems and structures. Many excellent books and articles elucidate the politics of self-care, including Kim and Schalk's "Reclaiming the Radical Politics of Self-Care: A Crip-of-Color Critique" and Hobart and Kneese's "Radical Care: Survival Strategies for Uncertain Times." Hobart and Kneese connect the ways in which "Care has reentered the zeitgeist. In the immediate aftermath of the 2016 US presidential election…. But for all the popular focus on self-care rituals, new collective movements have also emerged in which moral imperatives to act—to care—are a central driving force" (1). Both of these pieces critique mainstream, capitalist-centered models of self-care ("self-care is both a solution to and a symptom of the social deficits of late capitalism" Hobart and Kneese 2) and argue along these lines: "As people invested in sustainable social justice practices, we must work to develop, enact, share, and teach a radical politics of self-care, learning and following the lead of those who have had to work hardest for survival ['disabled women and femmes, especially disabled women and femmes of color' (338)] and resisting the allure of neoliberalism and capitalism within our care work" (Kim and Schalk 340). Both of these academic pieces are packed with radical insights, examples, and arguments that are far too rich and deep to detail here. Many of my students struggle with these radical critiques, in part because they are only beginning to unpack legacies of white supremacy. Their immediate survival needs, and their struggles to take care of themselves in the midst of uncaring systems and structures, are their entry point into conversations about collective care work and radical self-care. When we connect our individual struggles to the bigger picture, we begin to see that self-care is actually a part of collective care narratives and movements.

*

Yoga is often sold as an activity that calms and centers us (in addition to the workout). Staci K. Haines writes that "the goal of self-care can be presented as an ongoing, unchanging state of calm and 'well-being'" (366). Haines does not see this as possible, let alone as an example of self-care. In fact, that constant state of calm can be a tactic of avoidance and numbing. Susan Raffo writes about how we sometimes need to be *activated*. She writes, "Some kinds of deep cultural freezes or control states will never shift without agitation" (86). She is not arguing for the kind of agitation that we see at, for instance, a Trump rally, not the kind of agitation that is toward violence and unrest, but the kind that is toward positive change. "When we commit to agitation as much as settling, it gets easier to discern when action is needed and when it is time to wait, to feel, to notice" (86). This ability to discern, along with the ability to have and hold boundaries and a commitment to let go of perfectionism and productivity narratives, are some of the things that make self-care radical and transformative. But for most of us, radical self-care is not easy. Yoga makes self-care more accessible, but we still have to make the commitment to "the process of extending self-care outward and building a collective capacity for substantive political change" which is, Hobart and Kneese argue, "hard work" (7). We need to make more space for this work, within and beyond ourselves.

Making Space (in the Joints, in the Mind, in a Culture That Keeps Us Small)

Our joints manage a lot of pressure; they provide us with the ability to move in many directions. They also can become enflamed, stiff, and immobile. We don't think much about our joints—unless they cause us pain; then we can't help but think about them. Recently, in my study of the pelvic floor and pelvis, I was reminded that the sacrum is actually a joint. It is supposed to move and to help us move. We might not realize the mobility, or immobility, of this joint. I appreciate the mobility that comes from my joints and try to honor the function and help others notice what we might be holding in our joints and how we might make more space as we preserve or gain more mobility.

The hands and feet have lots of little parts, lots of joints—complexity and functionality—and are often overlooked. We feel our way through the world with our hands and feet. I try to include moments for smaller movements throughout class—ankles circles when the leg is lifted in down dog, wrist circles as we stand in warrior II, wrist stretches as we stand in warrior I or as we lie back in reclining butterfly. In yoga there are a variety of hand yoga poses—known as *mudras*. In short, connect any two or more fingers—but there are many variations. Some are quite complex. While there are certain qualities and meanings associated with these mudras, they are effective stretches and can also be focal points for meditation. Swami Saradananda's book, *Mudras for Modern Life*, is an excellent resource for learning more about both the practical and esoteric benefits of yoga mudras.

Yoga can help us access a bigger concept of space—making space to be in our bodies. This might be the literal space we make in our homes for our yoga practice or the space that we take up in the world. This space might also be the mental space we free up in our minds when we let unimportant or all-consuming thoughts drop away. As someone whose mind likes to latch onto troubling thoughts and spin and spin and spin them around, I have had a few moments where I have stopped that spinning and chosen to let go. I have, quite literally, felt the negative thoughts drop out of my head like a brick, making space for more productive and pleasant things ... like myself. And the more I have practiced yoga, the less I find my mind uselessly, anxiously spinning.

Making space in our joints, our bodies, and our minds, can also help us to recognize that space is a privilege and encourage us to be more conscious of how we can take up more space, or less space, depending upon our social location and cultural power. Women are often taught to take up less space, literally and figuratively, while men are conditioned to take up more space. Black, queer, and disabled people are taught that certain spaces don't belong to them and space (land) has been taken from indigenous Americans. We can make more space for those who are left out or pushed to the margins. We can remember that there is space for all of us.

Roll It Out

My favorite not-exactly yoga practice comes in the form of rolling a tennis ball—under the feet, under the back, on any part of the body that needs a release of tension. I've learned a variety of techniques from Bo Forbes and have seen these techniques extended into other yoga spaces and physical therapy practices as well. In my own practice—and in the workshops or retreats I offer—it is easy to get lost in this myofascial release/self-massage. I encourage you to investigate specific techniques, but the basic rules are simple: (1) If it feels good, do it. If not, don't do it. (2) Roll in the spaces between the bones, not on the bones directly. (3) Be gentle and remember that a little bit goes a long way. (4) Breathe. (5) Move on when one spot has had enough (learn to listen to your body and stop while it still feels good). Exploration and paying attention are key.

One of the most popular techniques I use in class targets the tension that so many of us carry in our upper-back and neck. We begin on our backs on the floor, placing a tennis ball under each trapezoid—those two little triangles of tension and pain at the top of the spine/base of the neck—adjusting as needed. Just letting gravity do all the work may be enough, but we can also wiggle or roll the balls down the back between the shoulder blades and the spine. Here's where we find a lot of crunchy adhesion of the fascia. Our gentle movement releases this tension. This practice can also be done against a wall for better control of the pressure.

I include Bo Forbes's "football" in almost every class—5 to 10 minutes of rolling the ball under each foot (one at a time! standing or seated) with as much pressure as feels good, in any pattern or no pattern at all. This is also an opportunity to talk about the fascia, the parasympathetic nervous system, and one of my favorite topics—the vagus nerve (more on this in the "Imagine" chapter). I often say some people fall in love with football immediately, for other people it might take a few times before they fall in love, and some people never fall in love with football. I don't know what's wrong with them (insert the opportunity for a little laughter), but to each their own! I've fallen even more in love with using the Naboso Neuro Ball, which I discovered in a somatosensory yoga training. It has little spikes and splits in half with a bonus ball inside. (Not all spiky balls are created equal!) I use the two halves while working at my desk, which keeps my feet stimulated and my body and mind more awake.

Foam rollers are also a nice tool for rolling out tension and there are many variations and varieties. Some can be very hard and some can be very soft. It's important to use the foam roller that feels good and not to just try to roll through the pain. While tennis balls pin point tight spots, foam rollers iron out. And, really, all we need is the earth beneath us. We might just press the back side of our body into the earth, wiggle or roll around, and use it as our own personal massage therapist. (This embodied practice is my favorite part of JourneyDance!)

Massage and Energy Healing

Massage is not a luxury. It is therapy. The price and connection to exclusive spaces like day spas and fancy hotels make massage seem like a luxury, but it should be part of any healthcare insurance program. The connections to sex scandals, exploited by the media, make massage seem like a lewd practice. Yoga has its own salacious connections in popular culture as women's bodies are sexualized. It is not a coincidence that women dominate both of these industries—as clients and as service providers. Massage and yoga are sexually exploited, like everything else in American culture; this doesn't change their fundamental value.

Massage is part of my regular healthcare routine in addition to chiropractic care. When Covid-19 prevented me from being able to see my massage therapist, I was fortunate to discover some self-massage techniques at a Sea Change Yogathon (on Zoom). Self-massage is a way to care for ourselves and to show ourselves love. Touching ourselves is a powerful healing technique. I include facial massage techniques into my yoga classes regularly, sometimes at the beginning of class and sometimes at the end. We hold a lot of tension in our faces. I have been amazed at the results from these techniques though there is no substitute for a visit to a massage therapist.

Massage therapy can help a variety of conditions and can also help people develop better body awareness. A good massage therapist will consult with you about what you are looking for and will check in with you during the massage to make sure that the amount of pressure they are using is okay. Like yoga, you should listen to your body and communicate your needs to the therapist. I have had several massages where I ended up bruised because I was too afraid to tell them that they were going too deep. Silence is not a good practice in this context! But it is also not unusual, no matter how much we know better. It is difficult to advocate for ourselves in situations where we feel vulnerable. The more we get to know our bodies and our body's needs, the better equipped we are to receive care that is healing rather than painful or traumatizing.

Reiki, Healing Touch, and craniosacral therapy are gentler

approaches to healing and may be used in conjunction with massage. My favorite massages have been a combination of deep tissue and craniosacral. Susan Raffo describes craniosacral therapy as "a dance between the contraction of membrane and the expansion of fluid" with the goal of helping to "support the body to find its balance within any given moment—on its own terms and at a speed that makes sense for its desire to change" (211). Beautiful. (She also provides historical context and imagines an alternate history for this healing modality.) Letting ourselves be touched—cared for by a trusted bodyworker—is not always easy, but it can be transformative.

Tapping

Tapping is a tool I always forget about and use only superficially and yet, it still works. Tapping, also known as the Emotional Freedom Technique, allows us to tap into our own healing powers (pun intended) by interrupting and resetting the signals between the body and the brain. The idea is that when we encounter emotions that overwhelm us, our bodies and minds will respond differently. If you are interested in Tapping as a treatment, it's always best to consult with an expert, or at least the internet.

I have found success with intermittent application of this technique. In short, repeat a positive affirmation as you lightly tap the following areas with your fingertips: top of the head, above the eyebrow, side of the eye, under the eyes, under the nose, on the chin, under the collarbone, below the outer arm (below the armpit), and the outside edge of the hand. Or, do this tapping without the positive affirmation. Notice what shifts.

There are also full body tapping techniques that target the meridian lines of the body, as understood and practiced in traditional Chinese medicine, and are different from EFT. (Just search "full body tapping"!) Some yoga instructors use these techniques as a warm-up. On one long cross-country car trip I did full-body tapping at almost every rest stop and it really helped to endure sitting still for so long. I wish I remembered to do this technique more often!

Sounds and Scents

The ways in which scents and sounds can impact our mind/body and emotions cannot be understated. Scents can bring us to a different time and place. A certain scent, or a certain sound, can soothe us while another can activate us. Combining sound healing and aromatherapy with yoga can enhance our practice. A sound bath, offered by a trained practitioner, is a whole body/mind/spirit healing opportunity.

Every night I use music as background noise while I sleep. I have a particular Meditative Mind video that I use almost every night that is 174 Hz and fades to a black screen. Sometimes I search YouTube and find a video that sounds right: theta waves, delta waves, different Solfeggio frequencies. Many YouTube videos last eight hours or more and some include colorful scenes and imagery or kaleidoscope shapes that shift. When I have taught in rooms with projectors I have used these videos as background along with the sounds. Meditation music is, of course, available in a variety of places where music is available. We can search around and find what we like and use it with or without physical postures or meditation.

Aromatherapy and the use of essential oils also holds much potential as an addition to yoga practice, or as a tool in our lives more generally. I enjoy lavender, eucalyptus, tea tree, and some mixed oils. There are plenty of resources we can consult to find out more about the power and potential of essential oil use. Essential oils can be very expensive, especially the high quality oils, which are ideal for serious use. Oils can be used in a diffuser or applied to the skin. Different scents have an array of associated qualities and connections, particularly to emotional states. (Lavender, for instance, is calming.) We should also be aware of the potential impact on other members of our households since some oils are toxic to pets and some can cause allergic reactions, or other negative responses.

An instructor should never use an oil in a class without asking permission of the people in the class first, but it does happen. So, this is yet another potential hazard to be aware of when you take yoga classes. Likewise, you may not be fond of the music an instructor uses during class and some kinds of music might ignite a trauma response. Some sounds just rub people the wrong way, for instance music with chimes makes me anxious. For others, birds chirping is disruptive or disturbing. Most instructors are open to feedback on the music they use and are willing to take requests.

Music Is Life

Music is integral to mental and physical wellness. There is a whole lot of science about the ways in which music positively impacts our minds and our bodies. (I have not even begun to explore this area of yoga with anything more than intuitive stumbling.) Any music that we like can shift our mood, and certain songs can help us heal heartbreak or remind us of our power. Beyoncé's *Lemonade* has gotten me through some hard times, and who could not feel empowered by Lizzo's *Cuz I Love You* album? As much as I love music + yoga, when Covid sent my yoga into the world of Zoom, and I did not have the tech savvy to make the music work, silence and my voice became the music. When I attended JourneyDance teacher training, I was introduced to Spotify and worlds of music cracked open as I was exposed to vastly different music than my well-worn iPod could imagine. On Spotify there is always more to discover—it is an endless rabbit hole. My eclectic tastes have exploded.

Some artists explicitly engage with yoga themes and traditions. MC Yogi fuses yoga and hip-hop and many ancient stories and symbols and Stic.Man (of Dead Prez) captures every essence of yoga philosophy in his song "Yoga Mat." CES Cru's song "Hustle and Meditate" brings a hard edge of intensity and Janelle Monáe's song "Yoga" is both play and critique. Plenty of artists create music that is intended for yoga and meditation practice. Some of my recently-discovered favorites include DJ Taz Rashid. I could listen to his song "Gold Flow" and the remix for hours on end. According to his bio on Spotify, "Taz envisions his work as being a channel for the expansion of global consciousness by giving his audiences a means to tap into their creative wisdom through movement, experience, surrender and awakening." Yes! Another favorite is Sol Rising, an independent artist and international touring DJ who combines "an eclectic mix of electronic music, mid-tempo, downtempo, chill-trap, ambient and lo-fi hip-hop." I don't know very much about genres or the technicalities of music and music production, but I know what moves me and I listen obsessively on repeat.

Music can become mantra—short phrases like inspirational quotes that can be repeated to help us refocus and remind us of what's important. Any song lyrics that speak to us can be repeated in our head or out loud to center and inspire us. Some of these songs give us not just a beat to keep us going or music to soothe us; many of them give us material for meditation or continued learning. For me, music is more about the lyrics, but I also vibe with the beat, rhythms, and feel of the song—the emotions evoked by the music behind the words. This can be dangerous when teaching yoga classes since some songs can evoke unforeseen emotions in participants.

Gail Parker tells a story about being in a fast-paced *vinyasa*-style class and the yoga teacher selected hip-hop music for the list that included the "n word." When she explained to the teacher how this made her feel, the teacher said she didn't hear it and apologized. The blind acceptance and subsequent avoidance of other students made the situation even more uncomfortable (46, *Restorative*; she further discusses this example in her other book, *Transforming*, in the "Forgiveness" chapter and epilogue). While it seems like an obvious act of ignorance and blindness that comes with privilege (I mean, *really?*, the "n word" in music for a yoga class?!), there might be arguments made regarding why we choose certain music and, maybe, choose to include music with the "n word," with the "a" ending. One argument I might make (though I would not use this music in a yoga class!) would be that it was the artist's choice to use this word and I am honoring their artistic choice. However, this requires forethought by the teacher and recognition and explanations as well as the opportunity for discussion. Clearly this teacher had not thought consciously about the music she was choosing to include. In my dance classes when I have "questionable" or "explicit" (or in the past, "not Y-friendly") language, I always call attention to it or talk over it loudly (or both). Sometimes I use the professor card and tell people that I am happy to talk more about my music choices after class.

In one of my classes, a student approached me afterward to say that hearing the word genocide had ripped her soul apart. I'll admit that I did not hear this word during class despite my familiarity with the song. I apologized and I explained that the word was used in a positive context, in an empowering and uplifting song about the struggles of young Black men to survive and thrive in urban environments (and there were no "n words" or "explicit" language in this song). She could not get over hearing the word itself. Fair enough. Most people don't come to yoga expecting to hear about genocide or other social injustices. Maybe they even come to yoga to escape such things! And yet, these are the realities of the world we live in. I didn't know what else to say in the moment. She was acting like a whiny, privileged, middle-class white woman who is just too delicate to hear things that are too much for her because she'd rather go about her life avoiding these topics. (I didn't say this! I couldn't say this! I shouldn't write this!) And yet, as a student reminded me: the right to comfort by avoidance is one of the most used escapes for white people and a pillar of white supremacy. If we aren't willing to challenge ourselves, we might just stumble into a situation that does the challenging for us. And this situation might as well be a yoga class where maybe we should expect to be exposed to ideas and experiences of other (and Othered) people. Unconventional yoga music can open up new paths of understanding, but it is also important to know who is in the room and what might activate someone. It is important to be sensitive to people's feelings and to be conscious of the choices that we make. But it is also important for us to offer a yoga experience that is in alignment with our purpose, path, and principles.

The American Yoga Creative/Critical Mixtape

We can branch out into yoga music that creates an opportunity to think about our practice in new ways—not just as background music and ambiance, but as American music that moves us in novel ways, adding context and depth. I offer my yoga mixtape, a compilation of songs that inspire my personal practice. They are generally organized from more upbeat and lively to more relaxing. This is not a playlist meant for practice ... unless you want it to be!

- "Hustle and Meditate" by CES Cru
- "Yoga" by Janelle Monáe (I come back to this song in the "Play" section, adding poetry and movement.)
- "Chakra Beat Box" by MC Yogi (In a training I learned some simple choreography that goes along with this song and with the sounds associated with the chakras.)
- "Inhale" by Common
- "River" by Bishop Briggs
- "Green Garden" by Laura Mulva
- "Stand Up" by Cynthia Erivo
- "Crimson and Clover" by Joan Jett
- "Yoga Mat" by Stic.Man from *The Workout*
- "When November Comes" by the Gorillaz
- "Volcano" by Damien Rice
- "Landslide" by Fleetwood Mac or Smashing Pumpkins
- "Love Song" by Adele
- "As Is" by Ani diFranco
- "As the World Turns" by Blackilicious
- "Heaven's Gonna Burn Your Eyes" by Thievery Corporation
- "Plastic Beach" by the Gorillaz, featuring Snoop Dog (my favorite song to do Bo Forbes's "football" to; play it twice, once for each foot!)
- "Mad World" by Tara MacLean
- "Everybody Wants to Rule the World" by Lorde
- "Love and Roses" by Janelle Monáe
- "32 Flavors" by Ani diFranco
- "Fade Into You" by Mazzy Star
- "Sweet Child of Mine" by Taken by Trees
- "I Don't Want to Think About It" by Wild Strawberries
- "Sweet Tides," by Thievery Corporation
- "Stardust" by Luscious Jackson
- "Listen to Your Heart" by Roxette
- "Water Pistol Man (Chocolate Mix)" by Spearhead
- "Farewell Wonkanites" by Primus and the Chocolate Factory
- "Damaged Coda" by Blonde Redhead
- "Imperfect Circle" by Jorja Smith
- "Willing to Fight" by Ani diFranco

Desk/Chair Yoga

Desk yoga and chair yoga are certainly a part of the American yoga scene. We spend a lot of time working, so yoga has to address this place where our bodies are often neglected. Sitting for long periods of time wreaks havoc on the body (and the mind!). Yoga can counteract these effects. Taking a few moments for yoga (stretching, breathing) while working at a desk can greatly reduce tight muscles and counter repetitive movements that can lead to other problems. Some people set a timer as a reminder to take a break. Some people listen to their bodies, which is not always easy to do when the mind is absorbed in a task that requires being glued to a computer. These simple stretches are suggestions for countering our time spent sitting:

- Alternately lift the heels and then lift the toes. Circle the ankles.
- Reach the arms up overhead and circle the wrists while taking slow, deep breaths.
- Clasp the hands behind the head, lift and open the chest and look up to the sky. Inhale and let the chest and lungs expand.
- Tilt the head to one side, reaching away with the opposite arm.
- Extend one arm, palm facing away. Place the other hand in front and push against (don't pull) one finger at a time to stretch the wrists.
- Scoot forward in your chair, hands on the thighs. Round and arch the back in a cat/cow.
- Lengthen the spine and twist to one side, hand on the back or side of the chair.
- Give yourself a hug (squeeze), hands on the shoulders (can gently press the shoulders down); sway or twist or find stillness. Switch the other arm on top and give yourself a second hug.
- Clasp one wrist, arms overhead and lengthen into a side stretch.
- Cross one ankle across the opposite thigh (or ankle or shin), open the knee (can lean forward to increase the hip stretch).

And most important: take deep breaths! Three deep breaths for each stretch is an ideal minimum, but even one is better than nothing. For added effect, inhale and lengthen and exhale and release. Inhale to open; exhale to return to center.

Chair yoga is a great alternative for people whose bodies cannot do the kind of yoga found in gyms and fancy studios. However, anyone and everyone can benefit from chair yoga.

Taking Yoga Outside: Hiking Yoga

Because we spend so much time at our desks and in our chairs (on our butts, to be more precise), taking our yoga outside can be a fun and playful way to enhance both yoga and time spent outdoors. Hiking yoga is a thing. I learned it at a Yoga Journal LIVE! conference in New York where we did Hiking Yoga in Central Park with Eric Kipp, but it is also just something you can do to complement any stroll, walk, hike, or backpacking trip. Both urban spaces and wilderness spaces—and all kinds of spaces in between—can be the perfect setting for some hiking yoga. I've offered Hiking Yoga on the Bangor (Maine) Waterfront, and through Downtown Bangor cityscapes, as well as along the river in the city of Odense, Denmark. I've also done my own Hiking Yoga on backpacking and hiking trips in more remote locations. In fact, complementing my backpacking and hiking with yoga has become a necessity! Here's a basic roadmap:

- Begin with some sweeping inhales and exhales—any yoga stretches or movements we would typically do to warm up. I usually do a few chair flows, a forward fold, a standing cat and cow, a side stretch.
- Then walk to another location. Perhaps there is a pre-determined space, or perhaps we stop at the next point that feels right. This stop might include some warriors—warrior I and II, side angle and reverse warrior.
- Then walk to the next location. Maybe the walking is done mindfully, relishing each step. Maybe we are with friends or family and we use that time to chat. Maybe we simply pay

attention to our breath and to the sounds of the environment around us.
- As we change locations we can also use what is available like a large rock or a railing along the edge of the trail or water. Perhaps this next stop includes some balance poses and standing stretches: a quad stretch that turns into dancer's pose, standing pigeon for a hip and glute stretch. If we have a solid railing, we can hang back and stretch the upper back. We can also do a pyramid stretch for the hamstrings, a calf stretch, and even a half moon balance.
- At any moment, we might bust out a tree pose standing by, or staring at, or placing a hand on an actual living tree! I often do unofficial poses that mimic statues or sculptures. When "The Good of the Hive," a bee mural that is a part of a worldwide project, was painted by artist, Matt Willey, in Bangor we did bee's breath in that location, gazing at the bees—a vibration connected with a bigger cause.
- Another stop might include a standing straddle stretch, triangle pose, and standing back bends. And then walk to another destination.

I like to end where we began—full circle. Some deep inhales and exhales, a forward fold (letting the arms hang and swing), a side stretch, a chest opener, and hug ourselves to stretch the upper back and shoulders. End with one final inhale and bring the hands to heart center.

Hiking Yoga is also an opportunity for an authentic practice of land acknowledgment—paying tribute to ancestors as well as contemporary indigenous peoples and movements. In my most recent incarnation, I chose an accessible route, in part to make the event more inclusive and to counter the inaccessibility of my fourth-floor space. Here's the event description:

> Take your yoga outdoors with a stroll through the urban landscape of downtown Bangor and its embedded natural features as well as its unique arts, culture, and community. Hiking yoga provides a sensory and collective experience, observing the sights, sounds, scents, and happenings along our accessible route. Social connections, histories

and hidden gems, embodied movement, conscious breath in the fresh air, and reverence and gratitude for the land where we live, work, love, grow, explore, and connect are all a part of this donation-based practice.

Donations will be accepted for the Spiral Goddess Collective Care Fund and Wabanaki Public Health & Wellness, an organization that provides a variety of programs and services toward healing land, community, culture, and the minds and bodies of Wabanaki people in and beyond Bangor.

The Things We Carry

Tim O'Brien's famous story about the Vietnam War reminds us of the literal and figurative weight of the things we carry. Some things are easier to carry. Some things are easier to set down than other things. We might easily let go of snide comments and hurt feelings, realizing that when we let these things fester they eat away at us from the inside out. But some things are heavier. We've carried them for years, maybe lifetimes.

In all of my academic classes I assign students "action" projects that can take on many shapes and applications of praxis—a fancy term for theory + practice. My students are brilliant and they have so many good ideas. One of my students proposed a project that involved getting together with friends and loading up their backpacks with rocks that symbolized the various different burdens that they carried in their lives. The rocks are concrete representations of psychic weight. They might even have words written or painted on them. Once the backpacks were loaded up, they would go for a hike. They would stop periodically and unburden their load by removing one of the rocks from their pack. After considering this rock, they would let it go. They would place it somewhere or even throw it out of their view. This activity could be done with symbolic rocks as well to avoid negative impacts on natural spaces. Other students have offered different versions of this idea. For instance, painting rocks with motivational pictures or words and then leaving these rocks in public spaces for other people to discover and be inspired by. Such rocks are great additions to community gardens and yards, or even to well-traveled walking paths or hiking trails. (This is not such a great idea in protected wilderness spaces!)

For my Embodied Social Justice course, I developed an activity that I call Picking Up Rocks/Clearing Our Path. After grounding and centering, I ask students to imagine their path stretched out, winding in front of them. In the first round we imagine our own individual path, moving rocks that are in our way—barriers to our growth and healing. In the second round we imagine our collective path—the big, seemingly immovable rocks of patriarchy, white supremacy, ableism, etc. We bend and lift and shift and find all of the ways possible to move these rocks out of our way, to clear the path toward the future we imagine together.

*

All of these tools are in our toolboxes and they will find us when we need them most. We will discover other tools as well. Yoga tools offer us play—a lighter form of practice—but first, we have to Imagine.

Three

Imagine

While I have always had an active and vivid imagination, I had never really thought about the connections between yoga and the imagination until I read the book *The Healing Power of the Breath*, gifted to me by a student in one of my yoga classes. In this book, Brown and Gerbarg describe how we use "imagination to move our breath and awareness to different parts of the body" (43). Taking the breath beyond the typical range of most people's automatic breathing requires imagination. In order to learn breathing techniques that expand the breath beyond the chest and upper lungs—down into the ribcage and into the lower body, into our whole body—we have to be able to imagine the breath moving to these other parts of the body. Imagination is a powerful muscle. Some of us have much stiffer imaginations; some of us flex our imagination as survival: disassociation or escapism or avoidance. For some of us, imagination is our more natural inclination; we can't help but imagine as we work, play, love, live, and breathe. Yoga plus imagination opens doors and makes new mind/body/spirit and community connections.

No yoga practice is complete without tapping into the imagination—not only the ability to harness stories or move our breath, but also to imagine ourselves as something bigger than ourselves, or smaller and less important than ourselves. Staci K. Haines describes imagination as "the ability to imagine positive and sustaining futures" (208). Positive futures are far easier to imagine than *sustaining* futures. She continues, "Imagining positive futures is vital for navigating violence, oppression, and systemic trauma" (208). If we can't imagine something different for ourselves, we might not be able to find our way out of the circumstances and systems we are stuck in. She points to writers and artists who imagine these futures "and then share that with the rest of us" (208). But, she argues, we need to ensure that "imagination is used as a practice of resilience rather than a practice of denial" (208). It might be difficult to tell the difference between avoidance and denial and resilience, but what we imagine is not only in our heads.

Our imaginations are often limited by the circumstances of the world that we live in. In her book, *Emergent Strategy*, adrienne maree brown describes the importance of imagination toward creating better futures and the ways in which "imagination is shaped by our entire life experience, our socialization, the concepts we are exposed to, where we fall in the global hierarchies of society" (17). She argues that "we are in an imagination battle" and that she often feels "trapped inside someone else's imagination" and she must "engage [her] own imagination in order to break free" (18). We are all trapped inside a world imagined by scarcity, exploitation, greed, corruption, and power-over systems. When we recognize the power of our imaginations—individually and collectively—we can not only work toward liberating our own mind/body/spirit, but also toward changing the narratives that shape our collective consciousness in limited and limiting ways.

Imagination is a valuable tool for understanding, integration, and transformation. In this final section, I explore a variety of incarnations of the imagination that take movements and ideas into and beyond the body, the mind, and the mind/body/spirit. We have to imagine the things that we cannot see with our eyes. We have to tap into our other senses. We have to imagine the things that aren't easily measured through the tools at our disposal or the powers of our conscious brains. This doesn't mean that these things are not *real*, it only means that they are more complicated than we might like them to be. We have to imagine possibilities for ourselves that are not constrained by the exploitative nature of our culture. We have to imagine the world we want to live in. We have to imagine what yoga can be.

To imagine is not to make up, but to tap into the vast personal and cultural reservoirs that we gather through our interactions with the world around us in order to "see" a new "image." Imagination is a creative endeavor, but not a blank canvas. When we see a tree, we might not see the roots—the vast systems and networks embedded in the earth below that tree—but we know that they are there. (And once they have been there for lifetimes, it is very difficult to pull them out of the ground.) As someone with a pretty active imagination and a love of science fiction, I am sometimes shocked by the rigidity and hostility of people with less flexible brains. Nothing in life is black and white; everything is complicated and messy. We cannot force or enforce one way of thinking or one way of being, or of one way of practicing yoga. Yoga—in its many incarnations—offers a path to play in these less visible realms. This play might initially frighten us, but we already play like this through stories.

Storytelling, Warriors, and Empathy

In (almost) every story there is the villain and the hero. In every good story, the villain is more complicated than evil and the hero is more flawed than the perfection we project onto them. In the stories we tell about ourselves, it can be easy to gloss over imperfections; it can be just as easy to dwell on those imperfections. We are hardwired to understand ourselves and the world around us through stories. Stories help us comprehend more easily and retain more information than we might otherwise be able to hold onto at any given moment. Some of our stories are really fucked up; it's amazing that we even survive. Some of our stories loop and weave; others get stuck on repeat. Some are waiting to be written. But all of our stories make room for imagination. Tapping into stories—ancient to contemporary, local to universal, archetypal to symbolic, personal to political, individual to communal—is one of yoga's powers. Another of yoga's powers is helping us to let go of stories that no longer serve us.

Myth and philosophy and history provide easy stories to pair and explore through yoga. Some yoga spaces invite in stories that originate in ancient yoga texts or in archetypes (like *The Bhagavad Gita* or stories about Ganesh, Parvati, or Shiva), stories considered to be primal and as old as humans themselves. Many stories offer lessons through interpretation. Some yoga spaces invite us to write our own stories. Writing workshops pair yoga and writing, fomenting creativity. Children's yoga is based around stories, a technique that adults can embrace as well. Storytelling brings all of our favorite stories to our yoga practice. Stories can be told through music, through movements, through symbols, through narrative—from history, from myth, from truth, and from fiction.

One of the most fitting stories told in yoga is of the warrior. The symbol and story of the warrior traverses ancient landscapes and yoga legends as well as contemporary stories of all kinds. The warrior is alive in our collective cultural imagination as well as in specific cultural contexts. Each incarnation of the warrior story can bring different dimensions to our understanding of yoga and our understanding of ourselves. Judith Orloff describes the "warriors of love" in her book *Thriving as an Empath: 365 Days of Self-Care for Sensitive People*. She writes, "We each have a mighty warrior within. This is the part of you that will fight for what you believe is right and guard you from injustices" (153). Here she connects social justice with the warrior, an aspect that often gets obscured by narratives of war and conquest. In the American yoga world, the focus on the warrior is often a masculine symbol or a symbol for veterans. But the warrior is also a social justice symbol, too often mocked by the political right. In an interview on *Anderson Cooper 360*, Cornel West said, "We've got a love that the world can't take away" and called for "love warriors," a sentiment he repeated at a Zoom event for the Department of Surgery at the University at Buffalo: "Love warriors are those who have decided to cut radically against the grain and attempt to engage in forms of care and concern for others. They are willing to give oneself, to emptying oneself, to give whatever gifts one has cultivated to make the world a better place" (qtd. in Hoffman). We certainly need more love warriors!

Tapping into warrior myths connects yoga with military symbols, veterans, and PTSD treatments. The men and women who serve our country, whose bodies and minds are often broken by circumstances beyond their control, are served by yoga's ability to foster healing for bodies and minds. Such healing can have positive reverberations into families and communities and into American culture more widely. Healing veterans' families and communities is a worthy cause, but it does not change the culture of war or the mechanisms of capitalism and imperialism. A stronger spiritual balm—and critical consciousness—is needed for structural transformations. We need more of these transformational warrior stories!

Orloff also connects the warrior quality to empaths: "Empaths are warriors of love. Once we claim our power, we are neither meek nor fragile. Our greatest strengths are our empathy and our desire to bring understanding to the world" (153). Empaths are often seen as being too sensitive and these sensitivities are seen as weaknesses rather than strengths. I was first introduced to the idea of being an empath in a fictional portrayal by my favorite author. Octavia Butler's protagonist in *Parable of the Sower* and *Parable of the Talents* is a kind of empath, a "Sharer," and she remarks more than once that her ability to share other people's pain is not a special power. However, many readers would disagree as we see the ways in which Lauren Olamina's empathy makes her a powerful leader and protector of her people. As Leah Lakshmi Piepzna-Samarasinha argues, "what is often missing from these discussions is how Lauren Olamina, Butler's Black, genderqueer teenage hero who leads her community out of the ashes and founds a new spirituality that embraces change as god, is disabled" (135). By imagining Olamina as disabled, her powers of hyperempathy are "disabled brilliance" that "makes her refuse to leave anyone behind, even when they are a pain in the ass or she disagrees with them" (135). Olamina is a warrior in this "Black disability justice narrative" (135). For Piepzna-Samarasinha, Olamina becomes a beacon of hope, noting that "we will leave no one behind as we roll, limp, stim, sign, and move in a million ways towards cocreating the decolonial living future" (135). Because Piepzna-Samarasinha identifies with this character, because she sees in Olamina the possibility of a future that is a "disabled dream," her empathy creates a new way for other people (like me) to frame Olamina and to imagine new possible futures as well. This kind of empathy, which taps into storytelling and imagination, is a different kind of hyperempathy. Orloff directs her readers in a way that speaks to Olamina's legacy: "As an empath warrior, nourish the peacefulness in yourself and heal the parts of you that are at war. ... May we see the humanness in all people, show mercy for one another, and have empathy for all" (153).

Being an empath is not the same as being empathetic. Empathy can be a cerebral understanding of a feeling of identification with another person. Our heart may go out to them, but we do not take on their pain. Empaths often absorb the negative (and positive) feelings of other people. It can be difficult to understand where we end and someone else begins. It can be difficult to understand boundaries, let alone establish boundaries, let alone hold boundaries. For some people boundaries are an obvious and taken-for-granted aspect of life, but for an empath, we might not even know boundaries are a thing that we are allowed to have. This was the case for me; I thought that boundaries were unfair to other people. I thought that if I had boundaries I would be selfish. Keeping other people out was not my way. It wasn't until I had a student who shredded her way through my lack of boundaries that I realized I needed them. It wasn't until I read feminist cultural critic, bell hooks' description of boundaries as something that we establish—not to keep others out, but to keep ourselves in—that I understood the importance of having boundaries. Before then, it had not even occurred to me that I was allowed to have a boundary; I did not even know what one was. But even with this understanding, I have struggled to have and hold boundaries. Sometimes boundaries are easier in my professional life, and sometimes they are much more challenging. In my personal life, I have come a long way, but there are always new boundary needs to explore.

My challenges with boundaries have been helped by finding resources that speak to me, sometimes before I even know I need these tools. Synchronicity, being in the right place at the right time, and other unexplained but seemingly fortuitous acts of the universe have helped me along in my journey of self-discovery as well as my yoga journey. One of the most startling instances of this was when I found myself in a "Yoga for Empaths" workshop with Bo Forbes. As she described the traits of an empath, tears silently streamed from my eyes, a release as a new layer of understanding bloomed. In only a few words, I was able to understand an aspect of myself more clearly. I felt seen and understood like I never had before. (And then a canceled flight led to me attending a day-long workshop.) This is also where I began to learn about boundaries in new ways and where I started to learn specific yoga techniques for helping to establish boundaries—from saying no with the body to using tennis balls for myofascial release work. But this discovery was only a beginning, and I continue to collect resources and tools that help me to understand and tap into my empathic qualities, to honor my intuition, but to also draw on logic, observation, experience, and reason.

Yoga helps this journey in so many ways, by offering tools of the body as well as the mind—the real world as well as the world of imagination and insight. Yoga heals and empowers empaths. But, really, it heals and empowers us all because, as Susan Raffo argues, "Please don't call yourself an empath as though this makes you different from others around you" (143). Raffo's point is important, but sometimes being empathic does make us different from others around us because in American culture we are conditioned not to feel connections to people or non-humans around us. We are shamed for being too sensitive, for being different than the accepted norm. Raffo notes that three different "emotional tinges" come with proclamations of empath identity: neutral, some kind of overwhelm, or self-righteousness (140). She explains, "it's hard for me to hear this outside of the cultural shaping of U.S. exceptionalism" (140). Heard. The kind of self-righteousness that comes from these proclamations is often an excuse to withdraw from life around us or to capitalize on "a kind of elitism" (142). Raffo explains, "There is something so deeply capitalist, so intensely supremacist, about turning the normalcy of life into something special, something unique…" (142). American culture drives us to try to find something that is unique and special, something that makes us stand out, or gives us a competitive edge. We are trained in individualism, perfectionism, and (white) supremacy.

We are all culturally conditioned in these systems, but the most striking aspect of Raffo's argument is the connection between what we might name as "empathic" and the impact of "highly activated trauma" (142). This connection adds a whole other layer to our naming of ourselves as Empath. She explains, "Highly activated trauma means that we can get quickly overwhelmed by the stimulus of other people's feelings. Literally, our emotional physical selves are full" (142). Trauma is all too common in the power-over culture of the U.S., as Raffo explains: "Domination culture is going to keep ramping up the trauma individually and collectively. It is how these systems function" (143). Teasing out the difference between empathic feelings and highly activated trauma is, perhaps, important not only for our individual healing, but for transformation of American culture's "domination culture." Thus, if we consider our self to be an empath, perhaps this is a call to something bigger than we are, not just "to get the support we need to integrate the trauma that we carry so that we are not in a feedback loop of overwhelm" (143), but to connect to and nurture "the rampant expression of life" (143). Being able to connect with and feel that rampant expression is a tool for Love Warriors. It is a tool that we should help to make more accessible to others instead of using it as a title, a trait, or an excuse for disengagement.

If being an empath is "not an identity, not a struggle, not a burden that some people have to bear. It's about being alive" (140), then yoga can help us feel more alive. It can help us to heal. Yoga can help us to connect with ourselves and each other, and it can give us spaces to explore. Stories can grow empathy, especially when we embody them.

Woman Warriors

When we tell warrior stories about healing and empowerment, we can rewrite warrior narratives in yoga spaces and repurpose warrior poses toward social justice. In a workshop I offer, we consider the ways in which history tells us different stories of warriors—of woman warriors—that cross cultures and time periods. As one online compendium notes, woman warriors of the past were fighting back against a male-dominated world. Their physical and mental strength were evidence of women's ability to lead armies, if not also nations (Redmond). Some places in the world have already heard this message loud and clear and have long traditions of female leaders in government and beyond. The U.S. is woefully behind the times. After the 2018 elections, we (again) wondered if this was finally the "Year of the Woman." Meanwhile, Woman Warriors like the Apache warrior, Lozen; the warrior queen of the Middle East, Zenobia; The Vietnamese warrior, Lady Triệu; the Irish pirate, Grace O'Malley; and the French entertainer and famous bisexual, Julie d'Aubigny all have unique stories that diversify the many masculine warrior narratives that dominate this historical and contemporary figure and cultural symbol.

The woman warriors of literature and popular culture also give us other warrior stories that can empower us: Wonder Woman; Katniss Everdeen (of *The Hunger Games* books and films); Xena the Warrior Princess; Eowyn from *The Lord of the Rings* universe (books and films); Nakia, Shuri, and Okaye from the *Black Panther* blockbuster films; Nanisca, Nawi, and Izogie from *The Woman King*; and the women from the films *Crouching Tiger Hidden Dragon* or *Kill Bill*, are only some of our inspirational on-screen warrior heroes. Some of these girls and women live to empower us beyond the screen like the powerful symbol of the Girl on Fire that I write about and teach about and bring to yoga workshops and mind/body dance fitness spaces. Wonder Woman's 2017 film also brought to life the real-world warrior, Swedish kickboxing champion, Madeleine Vall Beijner, who portrays Captain Egeria, Wonder Woman's First Captain of the Guard. Vall Beijner's story about how she almost literally killed herself as an athlete illustrates the dangers of pushing one's body beyond its limits as well as the ways in which a woman warrior can find a second life on film. The women of *Black Panther* almost stole the show in the first film and became the central focus in the second film. After Chadwick Boseman's tragic real-life death, the women had to carry *Wakanda Forever*. Fiction and reality intertwine in so many of our warrior stories.

Maxine Hong Kingston's memoir (*The Woman Warrior: Memoir of a Girlhood Among Ghosts*) can give us different ways of thinking about the warrior poses that show up in so many yoga spaces. The trauma of a "girlhood among ghosts" speaks to intergenerational traumas that are also explored in cutting edge fields like epigenetics. Kingston's woman warrior is not literally fighting bloody battles—she is fighting for identity and acceptance, caught between two worlds as an Asian American. She cannot simply sit back and expect to be accepted, let alone valued. She has to take action and make her own world: "In a time of destruction, [she has to] create something." Kingston's woman warrior also embodies the cultural power of Kingston herself who reminds us: "We're all under the same sky and walk the same earth; we're alive together during the same moment." When we tell these kinds of warrior stories in yoga spaces and sequences, we tap into the power of empathy that extends across time and space.

The Subtle Body: Energy and the Chakras

Many aspects of yoga extend across time and space like the elements of yoga that make cynics and skeptics cringe, roll their eyes, or roll up their yoga mats. I used to be that kind of yoga participant, assigning talk of chakras to a category of woo-woo that made me tune out. Again, imagination (and an open mind) are key to understanding these concepts, even if we don't accept them into our lives, minds, or yoga practice. The chakras are tools to deepen our practice and better understand ourselves. Some yoga classes incorporate insights about chakras as centers of energy—or life force, or *prana*. Chakras might be described in terms that sound rather vague and woo-woo. However, as airy as the concept might sound, the seven primary chakras correspond to the structure of the nervous system and endocrine system as well as the bundles of nerves that gather along the spine, and there are other minor chakras throughout the body.

Yoga offers chakra cleansings and chakra balancing classes and workshops. They are a tool that we can use toward self-development and rather than see them as separate, we can imagine the interconnectedness of this internal rainbow. Because we cannot see the chakras with the ordinary eye or by scientific measurements, we have to imagine them and imagination is a powerful sense that connects us to the knowns and unknowns of the universe as well as our selves. Artistic imaginings and renderings paint a rainbow swirling throughout the body. We might connect this rainbow to the spectrum of white light that contains all of the colors of the rainbow. We might further imagine the associations of this spectrum of light with the spectrum of gender and sexuality and the symbolism of the rainbow flag.

We have assigned meaning to the chakras, functions to their flow, and impacts of their blockages. And we may be skeptical about the form, function, and meaning of chakras, but the idea of chakras aligns with ideas of meridians from Chinese medicine as well as contemporary scientific understandings of neuro-physiological functions. These echoes across cultures and systems of understanding speak to our common embodied experiences. Tons of information about the chakras can be found online and they are, like yoga, a tool that we can choose to use as it fits our practice and beliefs. For some more sensitive individuals, the colors associated with the chakras and the energy fields that surround us are not science fiction. Reiki and other healing arts tap into these energy fields that otherwise remain mostly hidden or obscured. Yoga can open us to deeper understanding of energy and insight, but it is not necessarily an automatic result. And if we fail to harness the tool of our imaginations, we are likely not able to tap into these aspects of yoga.

While there are many sources, variations, explanations, and associations, here's a basic breakdown of the seven chakras—offered as a starting point.

The Location of the Chakra	*Qualities Associated with the Chakra*	*Corresponding Color*
Base of the spine	Grounded, stable, solid, present	Red
Belly/sacrum, below the navel	Passionate, nurturing, creative, emotionally intelligent, embracing change	Orange
Base of the ribcage above the navel (solar plexus)	Confident, reliable, disciplined, strong sense of self	Yellow
The heart center	Love for self and others	Green
The base of the throat	Communication with self and others	Blue/turquoise
The brow center/3rd eye	Intuition, insight, imagination	Purple/indigo
Crown of the head	Connection to everything that is bigger than us	Violet/white

While I once was far more skeptical of the chakras and largely uninterested in this aspect of yoga, I have found the concepts, correlations, and explorations in this realm of yoga to be inspiring and enlivening. They help me to imagine what is happening in my body and they help me to imagine ways to shift my energy and connect with my inherent, embodied power.

*

One of the most popular and common associations we might hear to the chakras is to the third eye, associated with sight into spiritual realms. The idea of "third eye vision" plays a role in seeing beyond the present and below the surface and is often considered to be a mystical or esoteric concept. Some may fear what an opening of the third eye will do. Some may want to tap into the power of intuition and sight beyond the world we live in, beyond the cultural constructs that rule our lives—like *Third Eye Vision*—the title of the first studio album by the American hip-hop collective, Hieroglyphics. Founded in Oakland in the early 1990s by rapper Del the Funky Homosapien, this group's work is creative and imaginative. On the other hand, Third Eye Blind, an American rock band, also formed in the early 1990s in San Francisco, chose this name which signals a total lack of connection to the spiritual world and a focus on the material world. The pop-rock sound, "post-grunge" status, and the band's most well-known song, "Semi-Charmed Life" speak to the meaning of the band's name and its pop culture status. Hieroglyphics, on the other hand, are a collective that exist in relative obscurity with a loyal fan base. Their music is conscious, critical, inventive, and original. It's no surprise that the two examples map along racial difference, which maps along power and privilege. American culture celebrates the material, while the less tangible realms are where imagination and insight roam. American yoga maps along mainstream versions focused on the physical, as well as a vast array of other practices that challenge this one-dimensional version of yoga.

Flow

Flow is physical, energetic, and mental. Slow flow is my preferred yoga mode and approach to life. Flow can refer to the style of the yoga practice, or the physical movements, or the movement of breath or energy, but it also refers to the idea of being "in the zone." In terms of psychology, flow is the ability to lose oneself in a pleasurable practice—to lose track of time and space because we are so focused on the joy and pleasure of an activity. When we are in the flow, we may lose our outward focus or our attachment to ego. We might forget to be afraid of how we appear to others and whether we are being judged. Our mind and our body are in harmony. When we are in the flow we are, as Bruce Lee explained, like water. When our movements are synchronized, we flow together.

Classes described as "flow" (or *vinyasa*) can vary greatly in speed and approach. Many classes flow way too fast for my comfort zone—the breath comes too fast and shallow and the sequential movements lack natural transitions. "Finding your flow" is a cue that I often give in an attempt to make space to encourage participants to let go of using me as their lead and to find their own pace, breath, and movement. Finding this flow is also about finding the flow of life. Like so many yoga lessons, finding our own flow is so important to finding joy—to letting go of striving toward productivity, perfection, unwritten rules, and obligations.

In my ongoing self-study of what it means to be an empath, I have to remind myself to "see what the flow brings" (Orloff 7). While I am generally laid-back and have an easy time going with the flow, it is also difficult for me to let go of control. Flow reminds us that we are really just along for the ride. Change is the only constant in our universe, and to return to Octavia Butler's wisdom via her character, Lauren Olamina, we can only shape change. We cannot control it, no matter how much power we have. So, as every surfer ever has said, we can only ride the wave that's in front of us. Sometimes we just float, but sometimes we become the wave.

The Mind/Body/Brain and Neuroplasticity

Yoga enables us to be more neurologically flexible; it is not an automatic result of yoga, but yoga provides us with the tools if we are willing to work toward more mental flexibility. Yoga engages the mind and the body, the mind/body, and the mind/body/brain. It does not take much imagination to see the connections between the mind and the body via the brain. Science is mapping these more and more every day. The mind/body/brain element of yoga is both super-complicated and super-simple. We used to be taught that the brain developed up to a certain point in early adulthood and then it just stopped developing and growing. Everything we did to harm the brain, we were led to believe, would cause permanent damage. But we now know that this is not true. (All those brain cells you killed drinking beer or smoking pot are not, in fact, gone forever!) The brain can, quite literally build new neural pathways. Our plastic brains change and grow all the time and we have the capacity to participate in this process, not just through reading and doing crossword puzzles, but through dancing and doing yoga. In fact, some studies have shown that dancing is a far more powerful tool in fighting dementia than the brain games that are sold to us for such purposes. Certain kinds of yoga that provide opportunities for novel (new) movement are also effective in growing new pathways in our brains. Engaging the mind/body in mindful movement goes a long way toward nourishing our brains. Stepping outside our conditioned ways of moving has a powerful impact on our bodies and our minds. We can change our minds by changing our bodies and we can change our bodies by changing our minds.

The mind/body/brain connection and neuroplasticity also relate to our emotions and the regulation of our emotions via our mind and body. We feel our emotions in our bodies and our brain interprets and names these emotions. Some of us are better at feeling our emotions and some of us are better at recognizing and naming our feelings as emotions. (Some of us struggle to do both. I continue to work on both.) Yoga can help us on both fronts. Further, we often see that the patterns that are imprinted in our brains are also expressed in our bodies. It is not a coincidence, for instance, that a slumped posture with rounded shoulders and our chin shifted forward often correlates with depression (as well as neck and back pain). When we are anxious (or angry), we feel it in an increased heart rate and more shallow breathing. When we bring our spine, head, and neck into alignment and open our chests, we can counter a depressed mood.

When we slow our heart rate and lengthen and deepen our breath, we can reduce anxiety and deescalate anger. These are not magic pill cures, but they are effective and often immediate interventions that we can make to help ourselves feel better—maybe even better enough to seek the help of a mental health professional or a yoga therapist! (Check out the work of Bo Forbes and Amy Weintraub for a wealth of information and practices.) Yoga helps us to counter the stress we put on our bodies, minds, and emotions by simply living in our toxic culture. It helps us reshape our bodies and rewire our brains. And it helps us tap into the body's healing capacity, our protective nervous system and some physiological magic.

The Vagus Nerve

When I first learned about the vagus nerve, sometimes referred to as the wandering nerve, at a workshop with Bo Forbes, I imagined a beautiful vine of light weaving throughout the body, making connections where they are needed. Its path is measured and utilitarian, but it is also beautiful and mysterious. Yoga taps into the vagus nerve, which taps into the parasympathetic nervous system. There is science here. There is also a lot that cannot necessarily be measured by science—the secrets hidden deep in our physiology by the complexity of the human body as an organic machine that is sometimes well-oiled and sometimes full of faulty wires and disconnections.

The vagus nerve is the only cranial nerve that leaves the head and neck area and it sends 80 percent of the communications between the body and the brain. (The vagus nerve is more complicated, but I will keep it simple—American style!) Resmaa Menakem describes the vagus nerve as a "complex system of nerves [that] connect the brainstem, pharynx, heart, lungs, stomach, gut, and spine" (5). He notes that neuroscientists call it the vagus nerve, but that he calls it the "soul nerve." The vagus nerve, he explains, taps into our "felt sense of love, compassion, fear, grief, dread, sadness, loneliness, hope, empathy, anxiety, caring, disgust, despair, and many other things that make us human" (139). "When you have an emotional response," he continues, "that's your soul nerve at work" (139).

What makes us human are our emotional responses to the world around us, and all humans have emotional responses. Some of us are just better at the emotional intelligence and embodied sensing that it takes to understand what our emotions are signaling to our brains, and to other people.

The vagus nerve does not connect to our thinking brain, Menakem argues; it is outside deliberate conscious control, but "with some attention and patience, you *can* learn to work with your soul nerve" (140). The practices that he offers in his book—like humming, belly breathing, buzzing, slow rocking, rubbing our belly, 20s (joint circles), Om-ing, and singing/chanting aloud to ourselves—overlap with the practices that combine to create what we call yoga. As Menakem points out: "most of these practices are ancient" (140). Our ancestors understood their own bodies, he argues (as does Raffo), even if they were not aware of the biomechanical processes that we know today, and often practiced these techniques within families and communities.

These ancient practices are also explained by polyvagal theory (which I will not attempt to capture here, but Arielle Schwartz is a great source and entry point to Stephen Porges' work), as it elucidates the connections between breath and movement and the mind and body and the ways in which these tap into our natural healing systems and help us regulate our nervous system. Our own regulated nervous system is important for interacting with other people in our lives—family and friends and those we don't feel quite so friendly toward. Menakem argues, "when your body feels relaxed, open, settled, and in synch with other bodies, that's your soul nerve functioning" (139). Tapping into the vagus nerve through breath and movement and deep-tissue work is not a miracle cure-all, but it has some qualities that verge on magic. When I was first introduced to "football" by Bo Forbes, I immediately brought this myofascial release technique into my yoga classes. By rolling the ball under our foot with attention and gentle pressure, we can reduce pain and tap into self-healing. It's a popular self-massage technique, but it is more than just self-massage. The vagus nerve is the x-factor here, and combined with the breath it is powerful stuff. The deep-tissue work we can do with tennis balls can be transformative physically, mentally, and emotionally. Or it can be a physical massage. Again, that's the beauty of all yoga practices—they are accessible at a surface level, but we can always go deeper—literally and figuratively.

An understanding of the vagus nerve, the soul nerve, helps to put into perspective the power of yoga and the reasons why it can be an effective practice even if we are just going through the motions at our local gym. When we practice yoga consciously and consistently, imagine the possibilities!

Authenticity

While authenticity can be connected to discussions around cultural appropriation, it is also an important concept more generally in yoga. Yoga can be a path toward authenticity. For instance, the field of psychology points us toward our "higher self," our "true nature," or our authentic self, which are all about living our truths and may or may not be found via a spiritual journey. Authenticity might best be described as the ongoing journey to know ourselves without judgement and without ego. It might be accepting who we are, but not settling into the qualities that limit our potential. We can use any number of tools on this journey to find authenticity. Yoga meets us where we are and encourages us to go inside ourselves. We can balance our emotions, let go of our ego, and find a union of mind and body. We can explore mental and physical challenges. We can let go. We can find community and solitude. We can find ourselves—maybe even better versions of ourselves. While we might embrace the magical or mystical, authenticity is hard work. It is conscious work. It requires tuning in rather than tuning out.

Authenticity might be as simple as saying what we mean and meaning what we say. It may be about being present in our current lives, not being stuck in the past or striving toward the future. It might be showing up for a friend in need or showing up for ourselves when we are in need. Authenticity might mean being observant rather than judgmental. The problem with gauging authenticity is much like the problem of measuring cultural appropriation. Who is charged with saying what is or is not authentic? Who tells us when we have reached enlightenment? The answer, of course, is that there is no such thing as perfect authenticity—only the path, the process, the journey. When we try to be authentic, we also have to be vulnerable and both authenticity and vulnerability are difficult paths when cancel culture, judgment, and jealousy loom over everything we put out into the world.

In academia (and yoga) there's this thing called imposter syndrome—the constant fear of being seen as the fraud we really are. Not smart enough, not good enough, not close enough to dominant culture's expectations. While women, people of color, disabled people, and members of the LGBTQIA+ community are most impacted by this syndrome, it can be found all throughout the dog eat dog world of academia. In the world of yoga, it might feel like we don't belong because of a variety of bodily factors, levels of training, or attacks and assumptions from the yoga police. Competition breeds insecurity. American culture breeds competition. Yoga invites us in as we are—as imperfect and in process. Within authenticity there is room for errors and opportunities for growth.

Feminism and Yoga

Authenticity is also a challenge in the world of feminism where what it means to be a feminist, to think like a feminist, to live like a feminist, can vary immensely. And, yet, despite the ways in which feminism is misunderstood and used and abused, it is also simple. Feminism is the core belief in the equality and value of all human beings. It gets way more complicated, of course. But just like yoga is, at its core, conscious breathing, feminism is, at its core, conscious living. Feminism recognizes that we are more than our bodies. In the world, our bodies are ascribed meaning—our gender (and race) is socially constructed and given value. The value assigned to our bodies provides us with privilege while it also provides conditions for us to be exploited and oppressed. Our social and cultural value is superficial, but the impacts of exploitation and oppression seep into our deepest core. Likewise, the impact of ascribed privilege sets some of us up to think and act like we are bigger and better. Yoga reminds us of our true value, which is no more and no less than any other person. Yoga as a tool helps us keep ourselves in balance and in harmony with our fellow human beings. Feminism gives us similar tools, but feminism exists primarily to counter the destructive impacts of our patriarchal, misogynistic social and cultural structures. We might argue that yoga counters these destructive impacts of American social and cultural systems and structures. We need the tools of both yoga and feminism.

Like yoga, feminism has many different definitions and ways of practicing. Like yoga, when feminism is filtered through capitalism, it can veer far from its roots and core principles. Like yoga, when feminism is skewed toward the nefarious goals of a power-hungry individual, it can be used as a weapon to control others and wreak havoc and harm. Some versions of feminism are superficial and others are highly developed and delineated. Power feminism promises women can rise to power and bring other women along, pop feminism brings feminist messages into mainstream pop culture spaces, and being a "bad feminist," as Roxane Gay describes in her book of the same title, means that the contradictions inherent in feminism make it impossible to ever get it totally right. Feminism can be used to marginalize some types of women who are seen as distracting and detracting from a bigger agenda, goal, or idealized image. For instance, the feminist movement of the seventies pushed Black women and gay women (and gay Black women) to the margins in order to placate mainstream white supremacy. Today, mainstream feminists exclude transgender women in order to maintain an essentialist ideal of what a "woman" is. These problems are not problems with feminism itself; they are problems with the systems and structures in which feminism operates. Likewise, the image of yoga that focuses on svelte, young, white, hyper-flexible, beautiful bodies is not a problem with yoga, it is a problem with the ways in which yoga is confined within these larger structures of white supremacy, patriarchy, and capitalism.

So, what do we do if we want to dismantle poisonous systems and ideas? We keep chipping away at the structures, holding ourselves and our practices and ideologies to standards of social justice and authentic, balanced mind/body/spirit health. We build new systems and new ways of working together to change ourselves and our world. Yoga can be a way of practicing feminism and feminism can be practiced through yoga. We can be feminist yoga instructors and many topics that we find in women's studies classes can be explored through yoga—for instance, body image, women in business, patriarchal violence, global women's studies, movement, empowerment, self-care, and social justice. In my women's, gender, and sexuality studies classes I give students space to explore yoga through readings or through attending my yoga classes. Some students make profound connections between what they are learning in class about feminism and what they learn about themselves through yoga. Melanie Klein, Chelsea Roff, Carol Horton, Beth Barila, Becky Thompson, Jennifer Musial, and Chloe Diamond-Lenow and many other feminist scholars, writers, yoga teachers, and activists are making important connections between feminist theory and practice and yoga.

Becky Thompson offers yoga at academic conferences for the National Women's Studies Association and also has offered free Zoom yoga sessions to NWSA members. In an email, she writes: "There is a lovely link between practicing yoga and NWSA's attention to healing and transformation. Contemplative practices become a poetic antidote to noisy, chaotic times, making it possible for us to slow down the mental chatter and focus on what the body teaches us that goes deeper than words." Again, healing and transformation are linked together. Thompson categorizes yoga as a "contemplative practice," but we might also think of it as a healing modality. When the NWSA 2022 call for papers noted, "*The academy is changing, and we want our conference to reflect that change and amplify it!*," I followed Thompson's lead and proposed a JourneyDance class, which is also a "poetic antidote" that "goes deeper than words." But even when contemplative practices and healing modalities go deeper than words, words are an important inspiration to enhance and support our practices that focus on the body.

Black and White Feminism and Intersectionality: A Digression

Throughout this book about yoga, I share insights that have American roots but are not directly tied to yoga. One lens that shapes how I come to yoga is derived from how I came to feminism—through Black feminism. My digression here is a bit long-winded, but I hope it elucidates many of the threads that I have been weaving (critical consciousness, cultural appropriation, authenticity) and speaks to why we must be critically vigilant (a term I learned from bell hooks) as much as we must be understanding of the often meandering processes that bring each of us to yoga and each of us to feminism. But mostly, this digression is working toward the larger point about what Black feminism adds to the theory and practice (praxis) of yoga. For this digression we need to engage our imaginations in order to see the disparate threads weave together into a new pattern of understanding!

The feminism I knew growing up was my mother's (white) feminism that was sometimes shared intentionally (no, you cannot go see the new Andrew Dice Clay movie with your friends), but most often her conscious feminism was undercut unintentionally through hatred of her body, insecurity, lack of boundaries, low self-esteem, and through her willingness (and/or passion) to work long hours for little pay as a supplement to my father's salary from his "real" job as if her job were just a hobby. (For me and my mother, work feeds our souls and the boundaries between work and play blur. For my father, work is an obligation with inherent boundaries. This gendered dynamic is a function of white supremacist capitalist patriarchy.) My mother's feminism was firmly rooted in the space patriarchy carved out for women. Many white (and not white) feminists struggle with disconnect as we try to live feminism in a patriarchal world, and I inherited all of these legacies while not considering myself a feminist. My fractured feminist sensibility was a privilege and a curse, born of the struggles of first and second-wave feminists who paved the way doing the best they could. But the best they could often meant that Black feminists were pushed to the margins of mainstream feminism. Thus, when I consider the feminism of my mother, divorced from the insights of Black feminism, it only makes sense that the feminism I knew growing up—the white feminism of the American mainstream—is a shallow, incomplete, contradictory, and white-washed version of feminism.

When I went to college and read bell hooks' book, *Feminist*

Theory from Margin to Center, my nascent feminist world was rocked and my formal relationship to feminism began. At the time, and for a long time after, this brand of feminism was just feminism. I turned away from mainstream feminisms without realizing that the whiteness inherent in these feminisms was what I was turned off by. I accessed feminism from a context of comparative ethnic studies, namely Black feminism, Chicana feminism, and intersectionality. But, here, these were simply part of critical race theory (before this concept was a bad word) and my larger interests in cultural theory, cultural criticism, social movements, and oppositional consciousness. I still did not call myself a feminist and felt unwelcome at campus women's centers where I did not feel like I fit in. During my Ph.D. program, I was teaching a class called Intersections of Race, Class, Gender, and Sexuality, which was cross-listed with the women's studies department. Still, I didn't really think about the theories I was working with as *feminism*, probably because I had only found rejection in academic feminist spaces where different shades of feminism were not tolerated. I focused on the forest rather than the trees.

I didn't come back to feminism until I started teaching introductory classes in women's studies in the second-whitest state in the nation. I had to re-learn feminism through a different orientation—one that centered whiteness. Alongside discussions of (white) feminism, I have engaged students in Black feminist texts and Black feminist critiques of white feminism. For (white) students who have never really thought about sexism and patriarchy and who have never learned about feminism, we are starting at square one. Teaching about feminism from square one reoriented my relationship to feminism. I started calling myself a feminist and much of my work on my campus and at my university became centered around women and feminism as well as diversity and social justice. All of my classes, for the most part, were built from texts by Black authors and critics. This was what I knew, what I connected with, what moved me.

Because I am human, and white, and passionately interested in too many things, and working a job that takes and takes and takes until it threatens to break, I am still figuring things out. My engagement with tools and texts, like intersectionality and Black feminism, are far from perfect. In my book *Girls on Fire: Transformative*

Heroines in Young Adult Dystopian Literature, I argue for an interdisciplinary, intersectional lens for understanding this genre and call for more books by women of color about girls of color. And in this call, I realized *after the book was published*, I did a shitty job of explaining just what intersectionality is. My inattentiveness and shame was further driven home for me by a somewhat scathing review that called me out for not citing Kimberlé Crenshaw as the person who coined the term (and criticized the ample typos). While this critique was accurate, and perhaps fair, I felt that it was a critique grounded in reactionary feminist criticism, the default mode for many feminists who gain cultural capital by pointing out the failings of other feminists. Given the larger scope of my argument and the ground covered by my book, as well as my limited resources and lack of institutional support (not to mention personal struggles that impeded the process), I did the best that I could. As cultural critics we are trained to hone in on everything that we see wrong with the object of our critique. I get it. I have been just as guilty of jumping on an opportunity to expose whatever I see as wrong with someone else's argument through my critique—this is a cornerstone of academic publishing. However, it has become a standard nod to Black feminism to cite Crenshaw as if she coined this term in isolation, and Crenshaw was not where I learned about intersectionality.

I rarely cite Crenshaw, not because I am trying to disrespect her work, but because I came to the term and concept of intersectionality from a different route—from the work of Black feminists as described in the 1977 Combahee River Collective's Statement (and from bell hooks' concept of white supremacist capitalist patriarchy). The Statement almost immediately lays out a "general statement of [their] politics at the present time": "we are actively committed to struggling against racial, sexual, heterosexual, and class oppression, and see as our particular task the development of integrated analysis and practice based upon the fact that the major systems of oppression are interlocking" (qtd. in Taylor, K. 15). This statement within a Statement, and concept of "interlocking" oppressions, immediately resonated with me and became a foundation and touchstone for my work. And there was so much more to discover and resonate. Crenshaw's work is important, but it is part of a bigger whole that is often overlooked. Many important historical and contemporary texts and critics are lost in the overwhelming amount of resources that exponentially expand with academic conventions and digital archives.

And so, finally, this brings me to the bigger point of this digression (thanks for indulging me!). All kinds of people come to yoga without the larger context of the social and cultural forces that have shaped yoga, just as all kinds of people come to feminism without an understanding of the social and cultural contexts that have shaped this movement, philosophy, and field of study. We come to yoga without knowing that it is more than a physical practice that is offered as a workout alongside other classes at our local gym. We might be confused about why our yoga practice is so contentious, why we are being accused of cultural appropriation. Likewise, we stumble into feminism, as many of my students do, when they sign up for a humanities elective and take an introduction to women's studies class, or read a book or a blog or watch a TikTok video. Many of us came to feminism as a part of the 2020 Women's March. We wore our pink pussy hats with only the current crisis as context. (I did not march because I was too busy managing a PTSD-fueled break down—my personal crisis overwhelmed the larger crisis.) However we get there, we come to feminism and find that it brings the world into a new focus. For some of us, feminism helps us heal the wounds inflicted by patriarchy and it transforms our lives.

We come to yoga because our doctor suggests it or because we take a class and get hooked, and we find tools for tapping into a deeper understanding of ourselves and maybe we even find healing from the wounds inflicted by the white supremacist, capitalist, ableist, imperialist, patriarchy. Maybe we don't even know we have those wounds; maybe we don't understand the source of them. Maybe, through yoga, which begins as a physical practice with hidden mental, emotional, and spiritual benefits, we find transformation. And, so, if we get hung up on the limbs of the tree, picking each other apart for failure to cite the designated representative of an idea—whether it is Crenshaw and intersectionality or Patanjali and yoga—then we miss out on the bigger picture and the substance of an idea or practice that has many origins and many incarnations.

And here's where I ask that we engage our imagination

muscles—the wisdom that comes from Black women's experiences of interlocking oppressions, and from traditions of Black feminism, is wisdom that fuels arguments for self-care (as discussed earlier) and brings new dimensions to yoga in American contexts. This connection is not a part of yoga's roots from a "traditional" point of reference; and yet it is just as authentic as any other framing that we bring to yoga in our contemporary world. Neither Black feminism, nor yoga, belong to me—separately or together—but when I combine them together I find truth and understanding that is at the heart of my spirituality, practice, and purpose.

Black Feminism Is American Yoga

As I began to link yoga and social justice in my academic teaching and yoga practice, an immediate connection came through Black feminism and the theories, methods, and ideas generated from Black feminists' writing (which is often, or always, generated from their embodied experiences). More work on this link is being done by scholars, feminists, artists, and yoga teachers, though it is important to note that just because a Black woman is doing yoga, teaching yoga, or writing about yoga, this does not necessarily mean that she is also bringing "Black feminism" to this work, at least not consciously and purposefully. For instance, in Jessamyn Stanley's excellent (and fun!) book *Every Body Yoga: Let Go of Fear, Get on the Mat, Love Your Body,* she writes about how her mother was "part of the late–1980s wave of feminist mommies," (15) but this reference has more to do with her mother's approach to nutrition, embedded in Stanley's story about her life-long struggles with her weight. Her mother's feminism gets one more reference: "shortly after she returned home from an epic voyage to the Fourth World Conference on women in Beijing," her mother became very sick and, Stanley explains, "just like a lot of true food addicts, my complicated relationship with food was born out of a place of sadness, not celebration" (17). In many ways, Stanley's relationship to her mother's feminism is a lot like mine. Our mothers were powerfully influenced by feminism in college, which shaped their approaches to mothering (and perhaps in ways less visible to their daughters), but were not passed onto us as overt political legacies.

Even if Black feminism is not consciously included in Black women's approach to yoga, its influence is rooted deeply in all social justice spheres. Michelle Cassandra Johnson's work has roots in her racial identity; she describes college as the place where she became "keenly aware of oppression, racism and white supremacy" as she "stood somewhere between" the white students and the "Black Student Movement," feeling like she belonged to neither (xii). She describes the trajectory of her work as wanting to "merge body awareness and healing with psychotherapy and social justice work" (xiii), a trajectory that comes from her embodied experience in "a culture that is wedded to white supremacy," which led her to become a social worker (xiii) while "disconnect" from her body led her to "become a social justice activist" and "longing for liberation in [her] body and beyond led [her] to become a yogi" (xiii). All of these pieces have been shaped by legacies of Black feminism which are, like most feminist legacies, embedded in larger social justice struggles. Johnson's important work includes, for instance, attention to "language-gender assumptions" (61), white supremacy, and cultural appropriation, but *Black feminism* is a particular legacy in academia and social justice circles that provides important insights in the world of American yoga.

In the same email that I cite earlier from Becky Thompson, she quotes one of the most famous Black feminists of our time: "As Angela Davis has recently written, 'Yoga reminds us that without deep, abiding practices of self-care, there can be no radical social transformation'" (qtd. in NWSA). Linking self-care and healing to conscious breathing, singing/chanting, and meditation, have been practiced by oppressed peoples as survival strategies for healing and self-soothing long before we were calling this "yoga." As Resmaa Menakem illustrates in his book, *My Grandmother's Hands*: "All of these activities will seem familiar, which is exactly why I recommend them. They are family and communal strategies that African Americans have used for generations. They helped us and our ancestors to survive, remain resilient, settle our bodies, and alleviate trauma for hundreds of years" (191). I would not categorize this as a feminist text, yet there is at least one reason why the book is titled after his grandmother—women, in all racial and ethnic groups, have held the responsibility of caring for children and supporting growth and resilience from one generation to the next. And Black women have had to rely upon self-care practices to "stand tall, endure, and continue to lead full productive lives," (xiii) as Jana Long explains in her Foreword to Stephanie Y. Evans's *Black Women's Yoga History: Memoirs of Inner Peace*.

Jana Long, a co-founder of the Black Yoga Teachers Alliance (BYTA), speaks directly to this legacy in her short documentary, *The Uncommon Yogi: A History of Blacks and Yoga in the U.S.* (which reaches back to Black yogis of the 1920s) as well as in her Foreword to Evans's book, which she notes, "has revealed the healing and wellness practices of African American women ages fifty, seventy, and older" (xii), practices that "serve to inspire Black women to evolve, aspire, and ascend to a higher consciousness for living as healthy, wholesome, and productive beings" (xiii). Long argues that "we have a responsibility to identify, appreciate, incorporate, and disseminate the myriad self-care practices rooted in our history and the practices of our ancestors ... so that we can share this history and these practices with our daughters, and their daughters, and those to come in the future" (xii). And Evans's book is a thick, thorough, dense, and foundational body of work that speaks to legacies of yoga and Black feminism.

Evans explains how she produced her book under "stressful conditions" and "a denied sabbatical request" as well as the Covid-19 pandemic and the stress of being a department head, all of which made "completion of this project more crucial as well as more challenging" (204). She connects to the legacy of Patricia Hill Collins who wrote: "'I wrote [*Black Feminist Thought*] while fully immersed in ordinary activities that brought me into contact with a variety of African-Americans'" (qtd. in Evans 203). Collins's emphasis on the "everyday" is an important Black feminist-womanist concept that Evans connects to yoga and meditation as practices that we are encouraged to engage in as a part of our everyday lives (204). While Evans's larger point here is about the central role of the "everyday" in Black feminist-womanist approaches to scholarship, she also speaks to the ways in which many feminists (myself included) engage in scholarly labor—with little to no institutional support and as intimately connected to our everyday lives.

Linking our everyday lives to our scholarship and activist work, resonates with another foundational feminist concept that Evans also highlights—the "feminist phrase 'the personal is political'" (236). She first notes this phrase in relationship to Tina Turner who saw her need for liberation as *survival*, not as a feminist act of self-care. However, Evans argues (to my earlier point) that "not all women who advocate for their liberation name themselves as feminists" and can still "advance recognizably feminist principles" (236–7) without claiming the feminist moniker. On the other hand, Evans also links this phrase with the work of Audre Lorde, who most certainly did identify as a feminist and who advocated for the idea that "poetry is not a luxury" (342) as well as the idea that "self-care is both compassionate and political" (3). Evans argues that "wellness is not a luxury. It is a radical practice and speaks to a foundational understanding of feminist theory: the personal is political" (342). Thus, feminist theories, ideologies, and practices, as well as what Evans refers to as "historical wellness" and Africana yoga (365), undergird our contemporary understanding of yoga in America, directly and indirectly. "Black feminism, feminism, and womanism," Evans argues, "each fuel the modern mental health movement" (241). And the modern mental health movement leads us back to yoga.

Evans ultimately argues that "Black women's contemplative practices as African-influenced yoga principals ... are parallel to Indian systems of thought" (366) and "infinitely compatible" (367). What I have touched on here are only highlights of Evans's extensive body of work in *Black Women's Yoga History*, which connects African and Indian origins while also firmly planting African American history and feminism as foundational to American yoga.

*

So many of the elements in this Imagination section coalesce around the work of adrienne maree brown (amb), whose Black feminist work comes to yoga not through academic pipelines or the mental health field, but through her work as an activist and community organizer, facilitator, and mediator; amb writes about empathy, flow, imagination, feminism, authenticity, social justice and so much more in many of her books, most notably, *Emergent Strategy: Shaping Change, Changing Worlds*, as well as *Pleasure Activism: The Politics of Feeling Good*, and *Holding Change: The Way of Emergent Strategy Facilitation and Mediation*. In each of her books amb is unapologetic about who she is, where she is coming from, and why she has put that particular book out into the world. In *Emergent Strategy* she includes a section, "Ok, But Who Are You?," and gives a short description of herself, which includes: "auntie, sister, daughter, woe ['working on excellence' learned from rapper, Drake], writer, facilitator, coach, mentor, mediator, pleasure activist, sci-fi scholar, doula, healer, tarot reader, witch, cheerleader, singer, philosopher, queer Black multiracial lover of life living in Detroit" (29), and then a more detailed and nuanced description of how life, love, family, and work have shaped her approach, which includes the categories of pleasure activist, healer/doula, and writer/artist.

It is impossible to sum up what the book *Emergent Strategy* is all about—it is unique, revolutionary, eclectic, exploratory, insightful, and thought-provoking. This book and adrienne maree brown are beacons of hope for "those of us who wish to see a truly, radically different world" (12) and this is exactly who amb is speaking to in her work. She writes that we must "demand of ourselves the possibility that we are called to lead not from right to left, or from minority to majority, but from spirit towards liberation" (12). With this call, she writes, "I suppose it is time to come out as a spiritual leader, in my own way." And this way is both wise and humble: "Which means—everyone is my teacher" (12). *Emergent Strategy* is full of inspiration from social movement activists like Grace Lee Boggs and the visionary work of Octavia E. Butler, as well as science, philosophy, nature, somatics, and so much more. In the section "Spells and Practices for Emergent Strategy," she writes: "Emergent Strategy is about shifting the way we see and feel the world and each other. If we begin to understand ourselves as practice ground for transformation, we can transform the world" (191). In this section she speaks to her "practices" which include yoga and meditation, noting: "I love intentional periods of practice, daily practices, new practices, and even outgrowing practices" (192). She asks, "What are the practices you need to line your life up with your values and beliefs?" (192).

While I could quote endlessly from this book as it connects to creative/critical insights about American yoga, I hope that everyone will read this book and all of the other insights and wisdom that amb has to share with us. But here's one more taste, a quote that I like to read during meditation/final relaxation in yoga classes:

> Together we must move like waves. Have you observed the ocean? The waves are not the same over and over—each one is unique and responsive. The goal is not to repeat each other's motion, but to respond in whatever way feels right in *your* body. The waves we create are both continuous and a one-time occurrence. We must notice what it takes to respond well. How it feels to be in a body, in a whole—separate, aligned, cohesive. Critically connected [16].

This idea of critical connection (which is an idea passed on from Grace Lee Boggs) is key to an understanding of the many threads that weave the tapestry of American yoga. We have to imagine the ways in which contemporary authors and activists elucidate the ancient practices of yoga, making yoga more powerful in the present and our collectively imagined future.

The work of adrienne maree brown led me to discover Alexis Pauline Gumbs, first through her book, *Undrowned: Black Feminist Lessons from Marine Mammals*. When I read this book, I used it as a tool for meditation. Each section provides deep insights into a variety of Black feminist themes like listen, breathe, be present, honor your boundaries, end capitalism, go deep, stay black, and slow down, but it was the following quote that opens the book that instantly resonated with me:

> What is the scale of breathing? You put your hand on your individual chest as it rises and falters all day. But is that the scale of breathing? You share air and chemical exchange with everyone in the room, everyone you pass by today. Is the scale of breathing within one species? All animals participate in this exchange of release or continued life. But not without the plants. The plants in their inverse process, release what we need, take what we give without being asked. And the planet, wrapped in ocean breathing, breathing into sky. What is the scale of breathing? You are part of it now. You are not alone [1].

This is a quote that I immediately began reading during meditation/final relaxation in my yoga classes. It speaks to the collective act of breathing that reverberates from the individual to the global and brings novel ideas to our yoga practice. To say that Gumbs's work is brilliant would be an understatement. The concept of "a guide to undrowning" and the ways in which she connects Black feminist lessons to marine mammals is creative, innovative, and enlightening. Throughout, she asks compelling questions, like: "What could it mean to be present with each other across time and space and difference?" (67) and "What becomes possible when we are immersed in the queerness of forms of life that dominant systems cannot chart, reward, or even understand?" (109). The last chapter includes activities as both a "Solo Version" and a "Pod/Squad Version." While not *yoga*, this book complements and extends yoga via Black feminism.

Finally, because I have already shamelessly mentioned Octavia E. Butler throughout this book, I will note that both adrienne maree brown and Alexis Pauline Gumbs have been highly influenced by the work of Octavia Butler. In my Spiral Goddess Collective space (and previously in my living room/Zoom yoga space) I have a print of Gumbs's artwork—a collage of Octavia Butler, only one of many collages of influential Black feminists that she has created (check them out on her website!). And amb is quite possibly the only other human being who shamelessly cites Octavia Butler more often than I do, linking her to what she calls "'science fictional behavior'—being concerned with the way our actions and beliefs now, today, will shape the future, tomorrow, the next generations" (16). I am convinced that amb is my much cooler sister from another mother. In an unpublished book that I wrote in the months after I graduated from college (early 1998), I wrote about a similar concept of the "science-fictional future" that argued that science fiction TV shows like *Star Trek: The Next Generation*, *The Outer Limits*, and *The X-Files* held the keys to a better future. If only I had been exposed to Octavia Butler back then; it would take me another decade to find her. Please don't wait that long. The ideas that Octavia Butler plays with, many of which are firmly rooted in Black feminism include crucial creative/critical insights for American yoga and beyond. As amb writes, "Octavia spent her life working through complex ideas of the future on behalf of humans" (17). We should all be grateful. We should all keep working through complex ideas, imagining better futures, and we should all care for ourselves and each other as a part of this process. Yoga is a tool for imagination and collective caring.

Yoga as Rest

In a culture that is focused on productivity and work as worth, we might have to imagine what it would mean to give ourselves a break. Can we step off the metaphorical (or real) treadmill and let ourselves just breathe and just be? Gail Parker explains this well:

> We live in a culture that places more value on doing than on being. We attach our worth to our accomplishments. We value how much we do, and how busy we are, more than what we do and how we do it.... Many of us associate being still with being lazy. We consider it a waste of time. Or we may worry that taking time to relax is selfish and end up feeling guilty. Sometimes we are afraid to be still because when we stop filling up every moment with activities, we encounter feelings and thoughts we'd rather avoid. Sometimes we are afraid to do nothing because our mind tells us we will never be able to realize our dreams if we take time out to be still [*Restorative* 171].

There are so many reasons why we struggle to just *be* rather than *do*. And when there is something wrong in our lives—whether it is a physical ailment or injury, a problem that needs to be solved, a friend or a family member in need—we often do something just so we can tell ourselves that we are *doing something*. But sometimes doing nothing is better than doing something. As Parker explains, "we engage in actions to make ourselves feel better and these are usually not actions that are best for the situation" (171). Instead, she suggests we reverse the common phrase of "'Don't just sit there, do something!'" to "'Don't just do something, sit there!'" (171). While Americans are notorious for being lazy, we're also good at making extra work for ourselves. But being still is not being lazy; it is a way of being alive and engaged.

Tricia Hersey, in her work with the social movement organization, The Nap Ministry (check out the memes!), and her book, *Rest*

Is Resistance: A Manifesto, takes the argument for the importance of rest to a structural level. She writes, "Grind culture has made us all into human machines, willing and ready to donate our lives to a capitalist system that thrives by placing profits over people" (7). The systems and structures of our society, culture, and world, and the institutions we work for, exploit our labor, set unhealthy expectations (often, but not always, from the top down), and kill us softly, so to speak. As argued in *The Care Manifesto*, "We are failing to challenge the limits being placed upon our caring capacities, practices and imaginations" (5). We are failing to flourish in our personal and professional lives because of the expectations of individualism, productivity, and grind culture. Hersey argues that "naps help you wake up" and calls for a collective approach to the problems of grind culture:

> Our collective rest will not be easy. All of culture is collaborating for us not to rest.... We are sleep-deprived because the system views us as machines, but.... Our bodies are sites of liberation.... There is synergy, interconnectedness, and deep communal healing within our rest movement. I believe rest, sleep, naps, daydreaming, and slowing down can help us all wake up to see the truth of ourselves. Rest is a healing portal to our deepest selves. Rest is care. Rest is radical [7].

At rest, our imaginations can engage with the possibilities of individual and systemic change in revolutionary ways. And yoga as a means toward deep practices of rest, relaxation, rejuvenation, and resourcing is another healing portal.

Because American yoga is so focused on the physical, we might also have to imagine how we can use yoga for rest. Many people struggle with *savasana*, the final relaxation portion of a yoga class, whether it is five minutes or fifteen minutes. Well into writing this book, I began to explore restorative yoga through books by Bo Forbes and Gail Parker. Like my initial dismissal of yoga as "just stretching," my initial dismissal of restorative yoga as just lying around doing nothing could not be further from the actual practice. My solo explorations were centered around Bo Forbes's question: "What would it be like if you consistently nurtured yourself?" She explains: "Restorative Yoga asks that you commit to the lost art of self-care.... Comfort and self-care are essential to truly support your emotional well-being ... add the support your body asks for" (163). Permission to literally and figuratively "add the support the body asks for" changed my perspective on practicing yoga, even though I had mostly always been gentle in my personal practice as well as my teaching. My quest to care for myself led me to share these practices with students and to sign up for YogaFit's four-day restorative yoga training instead of pushing forward on certification requirements.

In restorative yoga training, the practice was more centered around a couple of other questions Bo Forbes asks: "What do support and sustenance mean to you? How would it feel to allow someone or something to support you?" (163). Wait. Back up. Like a typical independent introvert, I glossed over these questions and focused on supporting myself by myself. I had to ask myself these questions, and still ask myself these questions. It is hard for me to imagine how it would feel to allow someone or something to support me. When I was getting ready to leave for Minneapolis to attend the restorative yoga training I was feeling anxious for a variety of reasons. My cat was not doing well and I knew I needed to take her to the vet. I had lined up a teenage neighbor to feed her, but I did not feel good about leaving her with no one who would care for her if necessary. The day before I left I had to do something I almost never do—I had to ask for help. I reached out to one of my cat-person friends who was more than happy to help me out. This was a big step for me and it took me into this training with the satisfaction that I had asked for someone to support me. In the training, we learned how to provide support for participants and in order to learn this, we had to learn how to ask for the support that we needed.

I learned this lesson again when I agreed to assist another instructor during her restorative yoga mini-retreat. I was exhausted, but I had committed myself to helping—helping, caring, and giving are etched into my bones. The group was relatively small and early on I attempted to assist the person next to me. But by the time I got there, she had already moved her bolsters to the other side. As I relocated her blanket, I quite literally watched my "helper self" walk out of the room and I knew I had nothing left to give. I settled into the practice instead. When I told this story, the instructor (who used to be my therapist) said, "you clearly needed to receive" and a lightbulb went off in my head. I can't keep giving all the time; at some point I need to let myself *receive*. I am sure I will learn this lesson again and will crave the opportunity to *receive* not only the benefits of restorative yoga, but to receive in other ways as well. Like many of my students and most of my friends, we find it easier to give than to receive. This orientation to ourselves and the world robs us of far more than rest.

Gail Parker describes restorative yoga, in short, as "restful and supported yoga" (177). Her longer explanation sheds more light:

> Restorative Yoga is a receptive form of yoga that requires no physical exertion. To avoid stimulating the nervous system and to minimize stress and tension, it is practiced in stillness. Props ... are used to support the body.... Breath is used to focus awareness and attention throughout the practice. The entire practice ... is designed to stimulate the parasympathetic nervous system ... [which] supports rest and recovery ... [71].

To practice restorative yoga, we need to be still and we need to stay still. This is not easy for most of us, but it gets easier with practice! To practice, we also need things to bolster us, which might be fancy yoga props like blocks and bolsters, but can also just as easily be the standard blankets, pillows, and towels that we use at home. (For some of us, investing in a yoga bolster might also help us invest in ourselves. I love my fancy yoga bolster!) We could all use more ways of practicing stillness, of "pushing a restart button" (177), of "recalibrating, repairing, and rejuvenating" (74). When we practice resting, we can be better versions of ourselves and live better lives. When we support rest as a collective practice, we can make the world a better place (all quotes from *Restorative*).

Stretching and Connecting Beyond Yoga

As my yoga journey continues to unfold, my mind/body/spirit has begun to explore a number of other practices and ideas that mesh with, extend, and deepen what I have learned through yoga. Even within yoga, it took many years of practice—and many more years of training and self-study and teaching and practicing—to begin to embrace ideas I never thought I would connect with. Yoga stretches our minds at least as much as our bodies, often in unexpected ways. So many people fear yoga because of their lack of physical flexibility. How many of us fear yoga because of the inflexibility of our minds? Both physical and mental flexibility can be eased into through yoga. We need to be open to new experiences in our bodies as much as we need to be open to new ideas and experiences of the mind. Yoga is one tool as well as just a starting point.

On my yoga journey I have discovered (and dabbled in) somatics, traditional Chinese medicine and Indian *Ayurveda*, Buddhist philosophy, qigong, meditation practices, mystics, neuroscience, trauma, embodiment, new ways of engaging with social justice, and so much more. I have found new ways of healing myself and engaging with my self and new ways of understanding different peoples, different practices, different traditions—all of which have moved me toward a greater understanding of the often flippant phrase heard in mainstream yoga spaces: we are all one. Believing that we are all connected is one thing; delving into those connections and connecting ourselves to people, ideas, places, and traditions that we have been taught are Other, is one of the opportunities that yoga provides.

When I took my first twenty hours of yoga teacher training, I had little to no interest in the philosophies of yoga and my first training had minimal inclusion of this aspect of yoga. Part of my disinterest was related to my lack of interest in religion and anything that reeked of the spiritual. As I continued my training, and as I was exposed to more elements from the other seven limbs of yoga beyond the physical practice, yoga philosophy began to resonate more with me. This small opening led to me being more open to a number of ideas and traditions that I had previously had little interest in. When I encountered the Rev. angel Kyodo williams in my work with The Embody Lab, I found myself becoming more interested in Buddhism, mostly because she made it interesting to me through her power and presence and through the ways that her presence and practice have challenged (white) American Buddhist spaces and practices. (And she reminded me of previous brushes with interest in Buddhism through the work of Ruth Ozeki, also a Zen Buddhist priest, particularly in her novel *A Tale for the Time Being*.) Pure gold pours out of the Rev. angel's mouth every time she speaks, or at least every time

I heard her speak! Even Zooming through my computer screen into my home office, the Rev. angel's presence was bigger than the room. I felt personally connected to her and felt like I already knew her. In that Zoom space, she held us all accountable regardless of identity or geographical location.

Jacoby Ballard brilliantly pairs Buddhism with yoga in *A Queer Dharma*; in fact one half of the book is about Buddhism and the other half is about yoga. And in Nityda Gessel's book, *Embodied Self-Awakening*, she draws together Buddhist practices, somatics, and yoga. While we need not lump together "Eastern" practices and juxtapose them with "Western" practices, the West can certainly learn from the age-old wisdom of civilizations that extend back 1000s of years. The U.S. is a baby and the least we can do is respect our elders as teachers and imagine new/old ways to be in this world as individuals, communities, and as a nation. As an infant nation we have ruled the world (or like to think we have) and we've done pretty well at fucking up the world (though we think we haven't). Our vision of ourselves as Americans must become cooperative and compassionate, humble and flexible.

Yoga is flexibility incarnate. Its ability to flex its influence across time and space demonstrates adaptability, growth, and evolution—all the best kinds of flexibility. Yoga meets colonization and appropriation by the West, generally, and by American cultural forces, specifically, with grace, patience, and an open heart. Yoga has never been one thing. It has been used and abused; it has been deepened and widened. It has been generously shared and closely guarded. When yoga becomes inflexible, it is no longer yoga at all. When we stretch our bodies, we might be better able to stretch our minds. When we balance our body/mind/and spirit, we might better balance all of the things that are thrown off kilter by the destructive ideas and practices of our white supremacist capitalist patriarchy.

Yoga as Remedy: The Pelvic Floor

Yoga can be a remedy for a number of physical ailments, mental challenges, emotional struggles, and spiritual crises—and all of these are interconnected. I can't begin to write about all of the ways in which yoga acts as a remedy—and there are plenty of books that consider yoga as medicine and/or tell stories (or share science) about yoga's healing properties. (For instance, Amy Weintraub's *Yoga for Depression*, which shares her story and other people's stories, as well as science to back it up!) But I need to write about yoga as a remedy for pelvic floor dysfunction. I need to tell a short version of my story and break the silence and shatter the shame that has lived in my body. And I have to imagine that my story can help other people.

The story of my pelvic floor dysfunction starts long before I recognized my "weak bladder" and unpredictable bowels as an issue, let alone as an issue with my pelvic floor. The more I learn about intergenerational trauma, the more I am certain that this story begins with my grandmother, and probably before her. I know that my mother struggled with pelvic floor dysfunction long before she sought treatment, but until recently there was only silence between us on this subject—until she had surgery and I started to get scared, and I started to get informed. But for at least 20 years before this moment of awakening and reckoning, I lived in ignorance of dysfunction (it was my norm) and I beat myself up—what right did I have to pelvic floor issues? I haven't had babies. Isn't that what causes incontinence? The shame compounded. My silence persisted.

When I finally decided to admit there might be a problem, books and internet articles were no help. Their message was the same as I had heard from a doctor years ago—do Kegels. Kegels are the remedy that a patriarchal system serves up for all women who suffer from pelvic floor issues. I worked up the nerve to try again and mentioned the problems to my doctor. The first time my doctor referred me to physical therapy, I didn't go. I was scared; I couldn't imagine what physical therapy might do for me. More than a year later I was referred to an Urologist who, again, offered physical therapy or medication or other options that did not sit well with me. I felt hopeless and helpless, but I compelled myself to follow through.

The first time I went to physical therapy, I started to panic and was about to leave when the therapist came to get me. Before she closed her door, I was crying. It wasn't the first time that she had faced a patient's tears. She was kind, but she was also ineffective, which I only found out several weeks later when she was suddenly replaced. Again, I almost left, but something stuck my feet to the floor. This new physical therapist was also a yoga teacher. She did not go right to the problem; she stepped back and took in the whole of my experience. She didn't shame me, and she listened to me. She discussed and strategized with me—she took a whole body approach. As Leslie Howard writes in her book, *Pelvic Liberation: Using Yoga, Self-Inquiry, and Breath Awareness for Pelvic Health*, "When the pelvic floor is off balance, everything on top of it—torso, shoulders, neck, head—and everything below it—groins, legs, feet—can be off balance. The pelvis provides a foundation and a fulcrum for our entire bodies" (2). This is not common knowledge; it is a well-kept secret.

The pelvic floor is complex and it is interconnected. The problems I was having with my ribcage and lower back were related. My diet was related. My lack of knowledge—of my body and *the* body—and my history of shame was related. And my experiences of sexual trauma were most certainly related. And Kegels were not the answer. One of the most important things that I learned is that it was not a lack of strength in my pelvic floor muscles; instead, it was that my pelvic floor was too tight. And this is the message and diagnosis that too few of us hear. Instead, we are told to do Kegels and the whole of patriarchal conceptualizations of the pelvis come to bear on our physical and mental health.

I wanted yoga to be the remedy, but the issue is not that simple. In fact, yoga can add to the problem; as Leslie Howard describes, she was doing "root lock" (*mula bandha*) so intensely that her pelvic floor got tighter and more dysfunctional. We don't know what we don't know until we know it, and most medical professionals, mental health practitioners, and yoga teachers have "misunderstood, or completely overlooked" or "underappreciated" the pelvic floor (2). Leslie Howard's book is a starting point toward understanding and appreciation. She explores anatomy as well as cultural myths and harmful practices—the physical and the mental—and she offers up yoga as part of a treatment plan.

I didn't find Leslie Howard's book until toward the end of my work with my physical therapist, Becca Mason, when I signed up for a YogaFit training (taught by a pelvic floor physical therapist, Alison

Presley). Becca changed my life and opened my eyes, and Alison reinforced my confidence and my ability to share wisdom about the pelvic floor with my students. One thing that both of these women have—besides a shared profession and passion for the pelvic floor—is the ability to speak frankly about our bodies and their functionality "down there." They vanquish shame and understand the complex interconnections of the human body/mind/spirit. They give us hope; and they give us practical tools that bring empowerment.

I am not cured, because there is no cure, but I am far better equipped to know and understand my body. I am able to adapt my habits, to pay attention to my body, and adjust my yoga practice toward a more functional body and a healthier pelvic floor. This is what the healthcare system—and yoga—should always offer us. Embodied knowledge and practice is the key to many other secrets that our bodies hold and many aspects of our bodies that we don't need to hide.

Embodied Yoga

For a long time I took the concept of embodiment for granted. I thought being in my body was a given, but I didn't realize how much I was not in my body until I found myself having a fight/flight reaction, only feeling safe huddling into the smallest space I could find (under my desk), crying uncontrollably, feeling like I was losing my mind and somehow also watching all of this from outside my body. Wow. It still took me too long to put the pieces together (PTSD, bitch!) and begin to put my pieces back together. I think I am getting better at staying in my body and noticing when I need to return to what the Rev. angel calls point (at the base of the belly). But what I am also learning is how completely disembodied most people are, and this realization is one reason why I wrote this book.

So, what does it mean to be embodied, to be in your body? That's not an easy question to answer. It has one of those frustrating answers of: you just know when you are. You have to feel it. Okay, totally not helpful, especially because we also might not know when we aren't embodied, which is the baseline state for most of us. So, what I can offer is some collected wisdom that we can reflect upon, starting with Susanna Barkataki who writes that "reflection is often the gateway to embodiment" (21). So, perhaps we are one step closer to embodiment through our reflection on the question of embodiment! If only it was that easy.

The Embody Lab describes embodiment as "a process of realizing each aspect of our self—feeling and experiencing its connection to the whole." And to embody is "to manifest—to make visible, tangible, and real." So, as we feel and experience each part of ourselves in connection to our whole self, then we are closer to embodiment. Or maybe it is easier to understand embodiment as its opposite: "As the unapologetic expression of that full self, embodiment can be understood as the antithesis of oppression." Oppression certainly keeps us from being able to feel whole, but perhaps we do not always feel our oppression as an embodied understanding. As Fariha Róisín writes in *Who Is Wellness For?: An Examination of Wellness Culture and Who It Leaves Behind*, "Embodiment is political, especially when many of us have been systematically disembodied on multiple fronts" (132). The fracturing of our wholeness by interlocking systems of oppression means that we are separated from each other as much as we are separated from ourselves. Jacoby Ballard writes that "we cannot be whole without being embodied, which is the wisdom and utility of yoga or any embodied practice" (185). So, perhaps the *practices* that help us be more embodied are ultimately the key to embodiment! By participating in embodied practices we might find what Nityda Gessel describes: "Embodiment is a grounded and calm sense of ease that allows us the capacity to open our hearts and pour compassion inward and outward" (5). Thus, embodiment is about being in our own bodies as well as being able to connect with other bodies.

Perhaps embodiment is something that we have to continually reinforce and reconnect to. It is never a given. It is never a permanent state. Our practices—like yoga, meditation, conscious dance—remind us to be in our body because it is so easy to leave our body when the going gets tough. So consciousness of ourselves in our bodies is key. Embodied awareness is, according to Gail Parker, "awareness that reaches deep into the nervous system, where contracted states caused by stress and trauma can release. This is where profound and lasting change takes place" (*Restorative* 187). Now we might be getting somewhere. Through our embodied practices, we get closer and closer to embodiment, we begin to perceive through embodied awareness. And this work is not easy. It takes time and consistent practice. And this work and practice, when done with the right tools, in the right combinations, at the right times, can lead to the profound and lasting change that Gail Parker refers to. Again, adrienne maree brown sheds light here via Generative Somatics: "'Embodied transformation is foundational change that shows in our actions, ways of being, relating, and perceiving. It is transformation that sustains over time." (qtd. in *Pleasure Activism* 17). So when we find that we are acting in our best interests, in alignment with our purpose, from embodied ways of knowing and understanding, perceiving and relating, then we can begin to understand that we are embodied. And maybe this understanding and this transformation begins with an unfamiliar sensation while practicing yoga or dance. Maybe the sensation is fleeting. As Gessel writes, "Without embodiment, we lose our connection to the present moment" (4). But once we have experienced the sensation, we can continue to practice and trust that we will recognize it when it comes again. Gessel continues, "With embodiment, we recognize our bodies, our hearts, as home" (5). And feeling embodied will come more often and we will hold onto the feeling longer and then we will find that it is just a part of us and we are embodied.

The good news is that yoga is a practice that leads to being more embodied—to being in the present moment and to feeling at home in our bodies—and we can access yoga in a few deep breaths, a few moments of stillness and breath, a few flowing postures; we don't have to have a strict one-hour class to achieve embodiment. We can further find embodiment during a swim in the ocean, a walk through the woods, a weight-lifting session. Yoga is a tool that helps us find embodiment in any practice—in all of the practices we enjoy. It is not simple or easy, but it is magical.

Yoga as Service and for Social Justice

Earlier I posed the idea that we might think about how service is integral to yoga. This is not a new idea. In fact, it is foundational to yoga, even if this aspect of yoga has been overshadowed by the gloss and glamour of American yoga. In *Living Your Yoga*, Judith Lasater writes, "So important is service that it has its own name within the system of yoga: *karma yoga*, or 'self-transcending action'" (129). As integral as service is to "the system of yoga," I think that Lasater overestimates humankind when she writes that "we are all inspired to serve the needs of others" (129). This might be putting a bit too much faith in human beings unless this inspiration to serve is qualified by Lasater's other argument that "choice is the heart of service" (129). There are plenty of people whose choice is to serve only those who meet a certain set of pre-qualifications, which are often thinking, looking, or acting a certain way. The U.S. welfare system, for instance, is designed based upon the very American model of helping others who we judge as willing to help themselves. Or, helping only the people who are "willing to work" for the help they receive. As individuals, and as a nation, we set certain parameters for what this willingness means, which often means that those who are most in need are left out in the cold, literally and figuratively. Lasater encourages us to "acknowledge the complexity of our motivation to help either when it is asked or because the desire has spontaneously arisen" (130) and she connects service to self-care, even though she does not use this word: "When you serve yourself, you make it possible to serve others" (131). Her book was published before "self-care" became a new way of arguing for "personal responsibility," after all.

In her book, *Sit Down to Rise Up: How Radical Self-Care Can Change the World*, Shelly Tygielski, the founder of Pandemic of Love, argues that "self-care and community care aren't mutually exclusive" (119). She describes a mutual aid model that "empowers community members to shape their own futures, helping to provide order and infrastructure to create the type of world we all want to live in" (180). Her arguments and examples are compelling and provide a very different approach to caring for others and being in service to others. She also provides examples of when some of the Pandemic of Love volunteers and some donors "resisted helping someone on the 'other side' of the political spectrum," which, of course, was common "in the months leading up to the 2020 presidential election" (191). The U.S. is starkly divided and only becoming more divided along arbitrary lines of left and right political affiliation. Our ability to serve and care across these lines is crucial for a better future for all of us, to state the obvious.

Tygielski's Pandemic of Love work started with a "spontaneous moment" and a Facebook post asking if anyone would be interested in joining her for a Sunday morning meditation (130). When the weather did not cooperate, she decided to "show up" anyway, and she continues to show up and the meditation gathering grows and grows and grows, leading to a "ripple effect" in and beyond her life and community. She explains, "We can create something out of nothing, and perhaps even more importantly, we can continue to cocreate as our actions ripple out" (148). (The idea of "something out of nothing" is a popular American concept brought to life most through the creation and growth of hip-hop. It is not the same as bootstraps theory.) She continues, "Rest assured, the ripples will continue to spread far and wide, but if you choose to deliberately ride or follow them, they will lead you to places beyond your imagination" (148). Radical self-care is a powerful variation on the self-care trend that functions as an arm of capitalism; only the radical leads to transformation. Yoga gives us tools to renew our energy and to practice self-care. We can follow these ripples into our service to our community and beyond.

*

When service grows into activism we move from the individual to the structural, from taking care of ourselves to taking care of the world. This is a big task, a collective task. It requires setting aside the ego, recognizing privilege, and reconciling the ways in which what we do impacts other people, other beings, and our environment— in intentional and unintentional ways. Yoga can help us take better care of ourselves and our families and can help stave off burn out for activists and care providers. Yoga connects communities and nurtures growth and transformation. Together, we can imagine a better world, and perhaps even discover tools and methods to work toward that better world. But there is not necessarily an easy and automatic connection between yoga and social justice. Like social justice and activism more generally, yoga for social justice involves inner and outer work.

Jivana Heyman writes about "Social Justice as a Practice" (140). He argues that "engaging in social justice as a yoga practitioner doesn't mean you need to get involved with every movement, nor does it mean that you have to be an expert at social justice. What it means is that you see social justice as a part of your yoga practice—something you *practice*, not something you perform or perfect" (140). In these ways, social justice is a complementary or corollary practice that, like yoga, can be about superficial performance or myths of perfection, but can also be about growth, enlightenment, and consciousness-raising. Heyman's advice to "step back and listen and learn from people who are directly impacted" and to find people to support and offer service to who are "already doing the work" is aimed at well-meaning white people and is on point. However, he falls into the same dichotomous trap of instructing people "from a marginalized group" to "also do your research," not to learn about different people's struggles and how we might support or offer service to people suffering from different incarnations of oppression, but to "find other leaders," to connect and find community, "and know you're not alone in the work" (141). White or straight or economically privileged people who want to work on themselves and who want to work toward social justice should also be encouraged to connect and find community, to know they are not alone in the work. Pushing back against tides of privilege is not easy, especially amidst the ignorance and misunderstanding of a growing number of "mainstream" Americans. And not every person who suffers from oppression is "doing the work" and maybe they don't need or want to be another leader. Maybe they just want to practice yoga. Assumptions about people's experiences and intentions on both sides of the oppression/privilege divide only further reinforce the differences that yoga potentially bridges.

The dichotomy is further reinforced as Heyman suggests the same practices of yoga toward different ends: to marginalized individuals he suggests *asana, pranyama*, and meditation to "build yourself up, to find strength, resilience, and joy, even in the midst of suffering" (141) while he suggests the same practices to those who he deems as not oppressed to "see yourself more clearly" and develop the resilience needed to "stand in the discomfort of the oppression that you may be creating in the world, or participating in" (141). If we all use these practices to see ourselves more clearly, to find strength and resilience and joy, and to stand in the discomfort of oppression, then we are standing together rather than on opposite sides of a culturally constructed divide.

Heyman provides the advice of "being open to learning," particularly if "you're not a member of a group directly impacted by a form of oppression" (140–1). We might argue that all of us should be open to learning about the similar and different struggles that we face, the similar and different ways that we suffer as a result of interlocking systems of oppression, and the ways that we can practice yoga and social justice together rather than giving different yoga instruction manuals to people based upon assumed privilege or assumed oppression. This might be one way of understanding the idea of union and the interconnectedness of all beings. We are all in this struggle to make the world a better place.

*

There are more and more programs growing that address particular needs in our communities. Here in Maine, Liberation Institute, co-founded by one of my students, Kevin Martin, and his mentors Piers and Jessica Kaniuka, is a non-profit that has provided yoga teacher training inside the Maine State Prison system, among other services in New England. Incarcerated men are able to gain skills but are also able to provide yoga to other justice-impacted men. Organizations like Sea Change Yoga in Portland, Maine, bring yoga to communities that have been impacted by trauma and not only don't have access to the glossy world of perfect yoga bodies and blissed out philosophies, but also have no interest in such versions of yoga. Vulnerable populations and marginalized peoples need yoga that is affordable and accessible and trauma-informed. But Sea Change also provides much more than physical practices of yoga under Elise Boyson's leadership. For instance, in periodic emails to the Sea Change listserve, Elise provides insights regarding current issues and how yoga relates, and can help us relate to, current events like the threat to *Roe v. Wade*. She writes:

> At Sea Change we're always asking how we can live our yoga off the mat and invite others to join us. In that spirit, I want to share why standing up for safe abortions is relevant to our mission. Ahimsa ... translates to non-violence, or living in a way which does not cause harm to ourselves or others.... Abortion bans perpetuate unjust systems and most deeply impact communities who already experience oppression and inequity, particularly Black, Indigenous, and People of Color, and people living in poverty.... Banning abortions in the U.S. would undoubtedly harm not just individual women, but generations of our communities already experiencing systemic disparate health outcomes.

Such statements are brave in a climate that wants to separate yoga from politics, as well as the larger climate where abortion is, perhaps, the most divisive subject of our times. It would be easy to interpret *ahimsa* as an argument not to abort babies, but Boyson dives into the complexity of this political hot topic. These are just a sample of the engaged and soulful work being done by individuals and collectives through sharing and spreading yoga. We can do more.

*

Yoga should not be a privilege even though it has largely grown and prospered in privileged spaces in the U.S. since the 1970s. Many yoga studios, schools, and teachers give back to their communities and this is a start. But simply doing yoga or donating to charities should not be confused with committing ourselves to the hard work of social justice. For all of us, the work involves understanding and unpacking our role and relationship to white supremacy (and other forms of oppression) and being less defensive. Those of us who are impacted by any or all of the interlocking systems of oppression can learn how to respond rather than react. Emotional dysregulation takes a physical and mental toll and nervous system regulation is a gift that yoga makes available to all of us. Being content in ourselves helps us to do this work and to find balance. As I have argued, the outward appearance of an individual, or their category of identity, do not imbue a person with an automatic understanding of systems and structures of oppression (repeated slights and injustice certainly do raise awareness!). Again, none of us is born "woke," despite the categories of identity that we are born into and maybe even despite the categories we choose to belong to. Many Black and indigenous and people of color are only beginning to unlearn the ways in which they have been conditioned by white supremacy because these are the norms of American culture and the myths that provide the promise of upward mobility.

Some choose not to take this journey. Most of us—or maybe all of us—are also still trying to understand how our fractured identities—our mix of privilege and oppression—take shape in this complex world. The insidious forces of white supremacist capitalist imperialist ableist patriarchy benefit from our ignorance and from our arrogance. Genuine curiosity, humility, and love must be met with patience and empathy. We are all complex, intersectional beings. The outside package only shows so much—words and actions are the measure of our contributions as we undertake social justice work. At the very least white people can be an alley (and an ally!) rather than a roadblock. Better yet, we can all be accomplices in the struggle. We all "Get in where [we] fit in," as rapper, Too Short, put it.

From Studio to Space: Reimagining the Business of Yoga

I am fortunate to have a career where I make a decent living. I can meet my humble needs and support my little family. This stability makes it possible for me to carve service into my life's work, and my job as a professor also comes with an expectation of service. The lines between work and pleasure and service have always blurred for me and I used to be much harder on myself about whether I was doing enough. I've come to be more accepting that I am doing what I can, and sharing my talents as a teacher of yoga and fitness/dance, healing arts and embodied social justice is, I remind myself, a substantial contribution. Whenever I can, I try to offer yoga, fitness/dance, and embodied social justice classes, workshops, and retreats for free. When I do make money (like when I was teaching at the YMCA for over a decade), I try to pay this money forward—toward my own trainings and toward opportunities for other women to take and teach yoga. I was in the process of setting up a scholarship and exploring the possibility of a non-profit centered around the idea of The Spiral Goddess Collective Care Fund, when an entirely unexpected opportunity emerged from the ether. Space.

For many of us, space is the barrier to our dreams of offering yoga, conscious dance, and other healing modalities to our communities. When I had the almost unfathomable opportunity to open my own space, I could not turn away from this dream that I never thought would come to fruition. When I walked into the space, it called to me. It felt like this space had been waiting for me. I did some rough math and figured if I taught about five classes a week and about five people paid about ten dollars each to attend, I could pay the rent. That was enough to get me to sign the lease. Initially, I was just looking for a space where I could teach JourneyDance. Instead, I found a space where I could teach all of the things that I wanted to teach. And I would have to teach all of the things to make ends meet. I could have just rolled out some yoga mats, as the building owner suggested, but the space called for something bigger, something more than just a yoga studio.

At the Spiral Goddess Collective, a Center for Mind/Body Movement in downtown Bangor, Maine, I teach yoga and JourneyDance and offer workshops and community events (and more). Perhaps more importantly, I create space for other people to do so as well. After years of having to play by the rules of spaces owned by corporations or nonprofits that operate with the same values as corporations, I was finally able to make up my own rules. But my rules don't mesh well with the needs that come with owning and operating a yoga studio—paying rent, operating expenses, and everything else that comes with keeping the doors open. My vision does not fit with the categories offered by Google Business and other platforms that serve business owners. I have had to learn a lot and I have struggled. I have had to employ all of my skills from writing and web design, to marketing and messaging, to interpersonal relations and mentoring, to organization and management. And more. There is always more. It is a collective in so many ways, but the ultimate responsibility falls on my shoulders. I have had to make hard decisions and I have had to enforce boundaries. I have had to ask for help. I have had to sacrifice time, energy, and aspects of my vision. I have had to accept that I can only do so much.

For the most part, my personal savings have funded this idealistic enterprise. I will likely never make back my initial and ongoing investments. The money I spend to ensure that the space and our offerings meet my vision is a part of my service to my community. All of the money that comes in via my offerings goes back into the business—the physical space, the scholarship program, the curators who offer their talents and support, and the micro and macro community. I have not yet paid myself for any of my teaching and some of the instructors opt to put some (or all) of their earnings back into this social justice oriented business. I pay out of pocket for help with cleaning and social media and other support work because I cannot do it all. I have made some relatively costly mistakes and intentional choices. And that's the most important thing about my "business"—it is, as much as I can make it so, *intentional*. I call the people who teach at The Spiral Goddess Collective curators, instead of instructors, because I see us as curating an experience through our offerings. I refer to it as a Center or a Space because, to me, studio connotes exclusivity and privilege, and I want it to be as open and as accessible as a fourth-floor space with no elevator can be. I call myself founder and lead curator because *owner* just doesn't feel right. I have been fortunate that my not-so-savvy stumbling has, so far, been a success—as far as mostly breaking even can be called a success. Money is not the only measure of success

The spirit of what I have created—the beautiful curated space, the trauma-informed offerings, the scholarship program and sliding scale/pay what you can pricing, and my energy, openness, and commitment—have attracted people who need this kind of space. The Spiral Goddess Collective merges all of my passions and dreams. In addition to what I provide through my unique offerings of yoga, conscious dance, and movement (with all the props that were never available to me in other spaces where I previously taught) and what I offer via the skills and gifts of other people (mostly women) in the space (yoga and yoga nidra, meditation, fitness and dance, sound baths, and so much more), I have created a space that includes: a Girls on Fire lending library with my personal collection of young adult dystopian fiction and feminist speculative fiction; My Sisters' Closet, a used clothing exchange; a resource center with books and materials about yoga and conscious dance; a feminist art collection; a ready supply of snacks, chaga tea, filtered water, and feminine hygiene products; a plethora of tarot and oracle card decks; a seating area for informal gatherings; and plants and lights and other inviting elements. The Spiral Goddess Collective is my offering to my community and to a vision of a world where we can all access education, embodiment, and empowerment. Where we can "Move and be Moved." It continues to grow intentionally and organically, and with a lot of labor of love but I can't personally finance this "heart-centered business" forever.

*

Some critics and pillars of the yoga and conscious dance community argue that we should not offer yoga or healing modalities for free (and often attach high prices to their offerings) because we are taking away from people who make their living through the same avenues. We should not undercut our value, especially because we invest a lot of time and money into training and planning and sharing our offerings. I understand the premise of these arguments, and I don't disagree. However, what I bring into the world for free is mostly being brought to people who cannot afford to pay for yoga or who would not otherwise do yoga if it wasn't free. Or, at least I am trying to create that possibility. At the Spiral Goddess Collective I have had to cut down on the free offerings and offer discounts and scholarships instead, though I still offer free yoga to community non-profits and UMA students. I have had to face the fact that my idealism does not mesh with the rules of the IRS or the "conflict of interest" policies of the UMaine system, a battle I continue to fight as my arguments are largely ignored by the powers that be.

My idealism also does not mesh with how people have been conditioned to consume. More than one friend in the business has told me that people will not commit to, or respect, my services unless they have to pay for them, that people devalue things that are free, that they have to invest in themselves. These arguments get in my head, making me wonder if I am mistaking martyrdom for access, if I am unable to ask for what I am worth. I want to offer something different than business as usual. I want to believe that another way is possible, especially when it comes to accessing healing, community connections, and transformation.

If we always have to make a profit, then we are always benefiting a system of haves and have nots. If we don't model a different way of being, we'll never change the ways we have been conditioned to be capitalist consumers. The thought of teaching only to those who can afford to pay me for my services breaks my heart. What I offer is of high value, but it comes with a modest price tag. People who can afford to pay for yoga and other healing modalities and embodied movement practices *should* pay, and I also ask them to pay for other people to do yoga too. Most people understand this dynamic and give what they can. Some people are generous with what they give. I don't judge and I don't ask for justifications. I know that what I do and how I do it could be considered "bad business," but it is good for my soul. I sleep better knowing that I am doing what little I can do with my power and privilege. I don't have all the answers and I am really just making it up as I go along, trying to balance a more than full-time job with my vision. I am not trying to suggest that I am better than other people who are making a living from their mind/body/spirit offerings. I am not trying to say that this model should work for every socially conscious business, but I hope that it might inspire other critically conscious people to use their power and privilege in the ways that they are able. We can imagine better ways of doing the business of yoga. And if we believe that yoga is for everybody, and that access to healing is a human right, then we have to find a wider reach. And, again, I have to be able to ask for help.

Yoga for Freedom

Freedom has many interpretations, including the contradiction between whether freedom means "freedom to" or "freedom from." In American culture we value our personal freedoms so much that we often seek such freedoms at the expense of others, and at the expense of the greater good and at our own expense as well. We see "socialism" as evil and dismiss collective change in favor of protecting what is ours—whether this is physical property or our families. America's vision of freedom is exemplified by the Covid-19 pandemic and our impatience with stay-at-home orders and masking. This pandemic has reshaped American life and the world of yoga. I've taken my community yoga classes online and have participated in a variety of yoga workshops and trainings in virtual spaces. This is freedom. And our freedoms are limited as the Supreme Court limits the rights we have—or don't have—over own bodies. Freedom is precarious. For some Americans being able to own as many guns as possible is freedom. To many others those very rights to gun ownership limit their freedom.

A common saying in the U.S. is that freedom isn't free. This phrase has been used by the right and the left, associated with Fannie Lou Hamer and uttered by Ronald Reagan in his inaugural speech. In a 2022 column, Naomi Law echoes these words and expands upon them: "My experiences tell me that Americans love freedom. We also believe that we are always right. Americans are comfortable making universal decisions and choices for ourselves and others. We believe that we are unquestionably wise. We feel that we, and those like us, deserve every available freedom." This kind of arrogance is what has helped to shape American yoga. We believe that we are free to make yoga whatever we want it to be and that we are wise, at least in part, because of the wisdom we have gleaned from the appropriation of yoga. The assumption of "those like us" have excluded all sorts of people from yoga spaces—from the South Asians and Indians that Barkataki defends, to the marginalized individuals and communities that Ballard references, to all of us who do not see ourselves represented in the images, advertisements, and spaces where yoga is bought and sold. American yoga is beginning to change—to hold itself accountable, but perhaps only because it can no longer feign ignorance. And accountability might have swung in the opposite direction, held hostage to cancel culture and superficial identity politics. I'm arguing that American yoga is something unique, with roots in ancient cultures, but shaped by some of the best, and worst, of what America has to offer. We are a young country; we're still growing up and American yoga will continue to evolve. We have a responsibility to critique and to shape it with critical consciousness and to practice it with humility and reverence as well as creativity and applications specific to our American contexts.

*

Yoga will continue to help us navigate our bodies and our minds, our lives and our dreams, and it will be an important tool in addressing the individual and collective trauma we experience in our lives and in our pursuits of the coveted and contested ideas and ideals of freedom. The freedom that yoga brings is a freedom of mind and body, a deeper understanding and a letting go. In *Living Your Yoga*, Judith Lasater describes how much she struggled with corpse pose (*savasana*) during her first yoga class, and many subsequent classes when she would "become painfully aware of how unrelenting [her] thoughts were" (58). Even when she learned to relax her body, her mind would be "charging around," creating "mental storms" (58). Many of us struggle with corpse pose. Because this is a problem that so many of us have, it makes sense to look to the bigger picture—the culture that we live in that keeps us constantly second-guessing ourselves, trying to fit in while trying to stand out, trying to accomplish everything on our to-do lists, trying to make ends meet. Our culture makes us relentlessly judgmental—of ourselves and of other people— but it keeps us pointing the finger at something other than ourselves. Lasater found that "as [she] studied and practiced more, [she] began to see that [an] emerging freedom from the tyranny of [her] thoughts was the only real freedom" (59). Freedom from the tyranny of our thoughts is, perhaps, the only freedom that yoga can provide. But we don't need to stop there.

After describing the ethical practices of Buddhism, Jacoby Ballard notes: "whatever we practice grows stronger. When we individually and collectively practice judgment, alienation, shame, and guilt, although these are inevitable and normal human emotions, we limit our freedom" (198). It is not about being right or being good, "as opposed to wrong or evil"; it is about bending "toward freedom" (198). There is freedom in letting go of the mental baggage that we carry; there is freedom in making space in our hearts and minds. There is freedom in creating a more just world. Larry Yang explains:

> True Freedom does not mean being in a place where there is no problem, struggle, or oppression. True Freedom means to be in the midst of those things, and still have clarity in our minds, openness in our hearts, and integrity in our actions. This is the kind of Freedom that will allow

us to move through even our most difficult struggles with greater effectiveness, ease, and benefit for us all [qtd. in Ballard 165].

Ultimately, I am arguing for the kind of freedom that is found through yoga that meets us where we are and provides us with things we might not have ever expected. This kind of yoga begins when we decide which aspects of yoga we want to explore further, which inevitably connects to other aspects of yoga. Our exploration might involve further reading and it might involve trying out new practices, or new perspectives on the practices we already engage in. Ultimately, as Gail Parker argues, "Freedom comes from within. As you begin to have embodied experiences of freedom, you can break the chains of your past and free yourself from cultural, social, psychological, and emotional tethers" (*Transforming* 67). Embodied experiences are few and far between unless we make the effort to engage in embodied practices as a regular part of our lives. When we engage in these embodied practices together, they are more powerful, and when these practices are informed by critical consciousness—when we connect our mind and body—we tap into individual and collective power.

Maybe we just want to do yoga and not have to think about it so much. I get it. I spend way too much time in my head (well, obviously, I did write *this* book!), but yoga has been part of my journey toward thinking less and feeling more, experiencing my life in my body at least as much as I do in my head. We should all think less sometimes, but we should all also think more sometimes. This is part of the life-long dance to find balance—balanced emotions, balanced expectations, and a balanced mind and body. With this balance, we are better prepared to find balance in the world outside of ourselves and maybe even to help create more balance in that world. With more balance, there is more freedom.

Yoga is one tool among many and it's worth having in our toolbox. So, take a deep breath, clear some space, and step into the possibilities because now it is time to play!

Four

Play

Yoga can be serious, but it can also be playful. It *should* be playful! Any activity that becomes stagnant, no matter how valuable generally or specifically, can become a chore and decrease its effectiveness. There are people who like predictable structure and there are people who like to dance to the beat of their own drum. Some of us move in the space between these two polarities. It can be difficult to get people to try a yoga class. It can be even more difficult to get them to try a dance class. Getting people to try a yoga class that includes dance—nearly impossible! People are afraid to be seen, to move, to cross boundaries into the unknown and the unscripted.

For many years I have taught dance and yoga classes that provide structure as well as freedom. Most people in a yoga or dance class want to be told what to do; it is not easy to break out of the boxes that we create for ourselves and that our toxic culture reinforces at every opportunity. But I keep providing the opportunities to do so. As much as possible, I encourage movement, joy, pleasure, creativity, exploration, and doing what feels good in the body in each moment. In my classes and programs I don't make promises about losing weight, burning calories, or shedding fat. Unfortunately, these promises speak to people's insecurities and external motivations for exercise. We chase myths and misinformation because that's what our quick-fix culture conditions us to do. I'm not delivering a "work out." I'm trying to teach embodiment and pleasure through movement within a bigger context of social and cultural transformation. Move, connect, and reflect. The "work out" is a side effect.

I have learned to become more unapologetic in my fitness-related teaching. Opening my own space to teach according to my values and principles has helped. I have to remind myself of this when I start thinking about how to meet the demands of the people and get them into the space. I have to let go of these demands and give people what they don't always know that they want or need.

When we *play* instead of *work*, we are challenging what Sonya Renee Taylor calls the Body Shame Industrial Complex. When we change the way we approach moving our bodies, when we find intrinsic motivations to move, we have the potential to change more than our bodies and more than our lives. We change our culture. This Play section—poems, bits, tools, insights, innovations, and activities—are starting points that I hope will lead us to other creative applications and explorations. Play, creativity, and innovation expand yoga's potential. We are transformed when we dare to let go.

Embracing and Exploring Yoga through Poetry

As a lover of words, I can't help but play with yoga in the realm of language and expression. This word play can take place in the form of journaling, sketching ideas, or forming experiences and feelings into words. Poetry is often seen as an elitist form of literature despite the fact that it has been foundational to American culture in a number of ways. It is elitist when it is tightly guarded as capital L literature, as high art instead of expression and play. The very American cultural phenomenon known as hip-hop is poetry (and then there's also hip-hop poetry!). Even the most obnoxiously shallow songs are poetry. No judgement. The sparse words, the bold images, the word play, the symbolism, the rhythm—all of these move us in ways unique, but not unlike, other forms of inspiration. Sometimes poetry speaks to us and moves us when we are least expecting it. What moves us is important to pay attention to.

Poetry speaks aspects of yoga that are harder to put into words. Susan Raffo writes that "the cells of the body communicate with us through poetry, through story, image, and metaphor. This is how we end up with a felt sense of something rather than only an intellectual understanding. This felt sense, this way of knowing from the body up, is how transformation takes place" (25). The felt sense of our bodies through yoga provides this "way of knowing from the body up"; thus, we might think about our yoga practice as poetry in motion.

I have used poetry in themed yoga classes for a local celebration of the humanities and I have a colleague who uses poetry to inspire social justice themes in her yoga community—in person and on social media. Many inspiring poems about yoga—and plenty not about yoga—can help us tap into new perspectives and ideas related to yoga and to life. Stic.man's "Yoga Mat" is one of my favorite yoga poems—a song about the metaphors that the yoga mat inspires. "She Let Go"—a poem by the Rev. Safire Rose, which can be found all over the internet—was introduced to me during a yoga training and I have brought it into some of my classes. When I use it in class I usually make the poem gender neutral, inserting *they* in the place of feminine pronouns. Such revisions are another form of play.

*

Some of the poems here originally appeared in my book *Women and Fitness in American Culture*; others have been written as I continue my yoga journey. Some of these poems reveal the ironies of American yoga and some delve below the surface of things. Some are light and fun and others are meant to get people to think more about themselves and their yoga practice. Are my poems *good*? Am I *good* at yoga? Neither of these questions are my concern here. Such questions are inspired by that competitive edge of American culture where we can't just be and we can't just be good; we have to be better. Yoga is—I'll say it again—a practice. Poetry is also a practice. Both are for process and processing. Gatekeeping and elitism have no place in culture or practice, let alone in play. Play moves us out of our comfort zones; we create new realms. We move and we are moved. We play and we grow.

*

In yoga classes and workshops, I love to play with the ideas in this poem, the literal and figurative meanings and practices of balance and flexibility—cornerstones of our expectations about yoga that tend to be more physical than metaphorical.

Balance & Flexibility

In life I find little balance
giving too much of myself
to too many worthy causes
Sacrificing sleep to work
relaxation to inspiration
Seeking a happy medium
between have to and want to

In life I have much flexibility
bending over backward
for anyone I love
or for expectations
Making adjustments
accommodating last-minute
changes and challenges
Stretching myself too thin....

In fitness classes
I have little flexibility
stretching toward my comfort zone
and beyond is mostly impossible
The push and pull refuse to give instead

Finding balance
stability with ease
Rooting myself
with purpose—
a foundation

—sometimes teetering
Always reaching....
then settling
for fitness and for life

This next poem came to me when I was thinking about how to describe some of the less tangible aspects of yoga. I find ideas about energy to be fascinating, even if they seem a little "woo-woo" sometimes! And yoga was the gateway to my deeper understanding of empathy and the challenges that come with being empathic.

Energy and Empathy

There are realms
Unknowable
Variable
Sensed and senseless
Sensation(al)

Paths without channels
Centers without solidity
Pulsing pairing
Emotion with sensation
With(in) self
From roots to ether

A feeling
Pushing on boundaries
Threatening sanity
Untethered
Tapping tools
Insight full (of) intuition

Embodied and
Imagined.

One thing that yoga gives us is new perspectives—on ourselves, on our lives, on our struggles, on the world around us. It's never a bad idea to see ourselves, our friends and family, our enemies, our country, and our world from different perspectives. And our perspective changes throughout our lifetimes and throughout our practice. Some days it is easy to keep everything in perspective and other days we lose perspective entirely. Like all things, perspective ebbs and flows and we adjust accordingly.

Perspective

Horizons set at the door
or in the back of the mind
A limitation without limits
A rise without fall

We might set horizons
As goals to achieve
We might forget that horizons
Are also setting suns

We may need horizons
To remind us of change
As our bodies age
And we push for a new plateau

We may need horizons
As safe points to gaze upon
As our bodies gauge
Distance and time

Horizons don't move
Body or mind

They are always in relation
In perspective
They are always still waiting
To be transformed
by Movement.

*

Ahimsa is one of the *yamas*—a yogic principle that shapes philosophy and practice. It means non-violence to ourselves and others, in thought and action; some of us extend this to animals and to the earth itself. I've been a vegetarian, more or less, since I was 13 years old when I became interested in animal rights. The problem was, I did not know how to be a vegetarian. Back in the day, and among my family and friends, it was a foreign concept. I did not know anyone else who was a vegetarian; it just felt like the right thing to do and be. The plethora of products for vegetarians and vegans did not exist, and I eventually started eating chicken and shrimp because those were the only two meats I liked enough to want to eat. The vegetarian options that exist today make it much easier to be vegan or vegetarian with little sacrifice. I was vegan for a while, but I am a lazy American who loves cheese and soft serve ice cream, and the non-dairy options for these aren't easy to find and just aren't the same.

While I don't consider myself to be more evolved and I don't argue that vegetarianism is a mandate of yoga, I do think Americans could eat a lot less meat. We could also treat the animals we eat, and the planet we live on, a lot better. We love some animals more than others. In India, cows are sacred; in the U.S., dogs and cats are family. What makes one form of life into food and another inedible? Of course, I could eat a lot less cheese, so maybe my dietary choices are no less harmful? I know the horrors of the dairy industry and I choose to mostly ignore them. Eventually, our individual and collective dietary choices will cause a reckoning (maybe they already have). I wrote this poem after a yoga training where the hypocrisy of preaching *ahimsa* was striking and comical, as many of our justifications tend to be.

Ahimsa *My Heart*

"Ahimsa," she explains:
"non-violence:
do no harm to yourself
or to others;
some think
this extends to the world,
to animals,
to a vegetarian diet."

I connect,
chasing *ahimsa,*
un/consciously violent
ideas turned against myself but—
doing no harm to others,
to animals,
compelled to eat
a strictly vegetarian diet.

"As much meat
as possible," she explains
her lunch order:
"it doesn't matter;
salad, sandwich
just pile
as much meat as possible
on top."

I comply, complicit,
sipping my smoothie and
decide to let go of
my self-violence,
let her hypocrisy slide,
round out *ahisma*
consciously,
humbly,
and whole.

Perhaps related to my love of food (as long as it is vegetarian!), I have struggled with body image in a variety of ways. Recently, I was struck by a social media post with pictures of fat women of every size and shape wearing black bathing suits. (To state the obvious, I use the word fat here as a descriptive term, not as a criticism.) The photographer framed the photo shoot as part of a bigger body positivity project. There seemed to be endless comments from women saying things like, "I wish I had known this was going on" and "I would have loved to participate in something like this." I don't know why I was surprised that so many fat women wanted to be photographed when they don't want to be seen *moving* their fat bodies in public spaces. In our highly visual society we see so many pictures of ourselves and sometimes spend countless hours filtering and editing and finding that perfect angle. Why wouldn't women want to participate in an event where they can come as they are (and put on a lot of make-up) and walk away with powerful, beautiful images? But what struck me, in addition to the number of people who commented, was how superficial "body positivity" can be. It is much more challenging to sell "fat acceptance," and even more challenging to get people on board with healing their wounds from the trauma inflicted by a racist, sexist, homophobic, ableist culture. (Our bodies hold trauma in all kinds of ways, including as fat.) We just want to capture an image that we can call beautiful and distribute widely. We want to *feel* beautiful.

Embodied movement can make us feel beautiful; it just lacks static visual proof. Yoga reminds us what our bodies can do and asks us not to get caught up by the things that our bodies can't do. But it goes deeper than the surface—or even the function—of the body. Yoga asks us to bring our whole selves, and this is what is beautiful. Side note: for the sake of play, there are many ways to read this next poem. Explore!

The Yoga Body (Beautiful)

Yoga bodies are not between,
not thick in the middle
not ample in the bosom
not brown or black or
crossing borders imposed
by gendered corsets

My body is not stamped
by yoga's standards
nor does it have the excess
or the access
to be able to claim
special status
as "curvy," as exotic
as hyper-flexible

[they say]
[defined
excessive
overflowing
off-white
walls
in minds
manifested in bodies]

[even when I stand
at the front of the room
some still wonder
who the imposter is
a yoga teacher she is

as Other
as   not]

Yoga bodies
are just bodies   [strangers
made real by movement   we can't know
grounded   without
expansive   connection
balanced   without
free   love]

Some spaces
are just bodies   [self/other
some minds   unhinged
are just spinning   creating
some worlds
are still
in the making
some bodies   all
dynamic   beautiful]

Found Poetry

Found poetry is one of my favorite activities; I use this practice in many of my academic classes to get students to think about a subject in new ways. A Found Poem is a new arrangement of words. There is no one way to create a found poem and there is no wrong way. (Except, some of my students who do not pay attention to the assignment criteria end up simply finding a poem that someone else has written and sharing it.) The Found Poem is a compilation of other people's words gathered from one source or a variety of sources. In many ways, found poetry is exactly what it sounds like: as you assemble a variety of found words, you find a poem. You make a whole from the scraps. Some found poems are simply words on a page, some are far more artistic and accompany drawing, painting, or collage. What's most important is playing with the source that is used to create the found poem and embracing and exploring the new interpretations we can discover by re-mixing a source or mixing a single voice with other voices.

The found poem brings new meaning, new shape, new perspectives. One approach can be to select random phrases from one book or one chapter of a book or from an article. Another approach is to select phrases from across a variety of texts. The "cut-up" method is credited to William Burroughs and was practiced by David Bowie and Kurt Cobain—literally cutting up paper into strips of words, phrases, and sentences and arranging and rearranging them. Maybe we select a few words or phrases from across our favorite books or from within our favorite book. Maybe the subject is yoga or maybe it is any one of infinite possibilities.

Another similar technique that my students have recently adopted is the blackout poem. In *Felon: Poems*, Reginald Dwayne Betts uses this technique as he blacks out words on court documents—the words that remain reveal truths, poetically. While the found poem extracts, rearranges, and reimagines, the blackout poem gets its power from what is left behind.

I love to assign found poems in my academic classes. Translating big ideas, feelings, and interpretations into poetry requires creativity and provides a different way of looking at a subject. It brings us freedom, insight, and playfulness. In addition to assigning found poems, I also create found poems from my students' work, to reflect back to them what they have learned as a collective. The following poem was pieced together from reflections that I asked nursing students to write about their yoga practice in my Integrative Healing Yoga class, an elective in the holistic nursing program. Many students had never done any yoga before taking this class. Their collective wisdom tells us much about what yoga is.

Yoga Is: A Found Poem
**From NUR 330 Yoga Practice Reflections,
Midterm Check-in Point, Fall 2021**

Yoga can be anything you choose to make of it
Flexibility
Strength
Relaxation
Meditation
Yoga is a little whisper to your soul to relax
Relax and invigorate, release tension
A tool to manage back pain
A coping mechanism
Shared time with your children
There's history and depth

Breath and movement
The thing you do to heal from exercise
To heal from trauma, from life
A focus on the breath
A connection within yourself
Lessening tension
Within your body—and deeper—
Within yourself
Yoga is a way of life (I used to say this with sarcasm;
Now I know it's true)
Mental, physical, and cultural health
The mind/body connections
The self in relation to the world
Teaching the body to be aware of its energy and potential
Realization and relaxation
A focus
A meditation in movement,
To transcend movement
To resonate
Within and beyond
If we choose to be open to the experience
Breathe into open passageways
Finding confidence and empowerment
Pay attention
And find healing

Move Your Yoga: Dance

Dance, with or without choreography, is another form of play. Like yoga and other mind/body practices, dance has been co-opted, contained, abused, used toward control—of one's own body or the bodies of others (and Others). But dance—in its infinite variations, origins, traditions—is just movement. It is movement, with or without music, with or without message, with or without intention. Every culture has a form of dance—spiritual, cultural, traditional—performed or used to process and connect. Like yoga, dance has been contained by the box of "fitness." So much of fitness is linear, mapped along the body's structure, functional lines of movement in one plane or another plane. So many people who work out are afraid to break out of this box. So much of yoga is mapped along the body in a similar way, contained by the official or traditional poses. The frozen moment in time is when perfection aligns. But movement breaks these chains. Dance is not so easily contained. Neither is yoga.

So many yoga poses require stillness, settling in, sinking, breathing. Again, yoga is super serious stuff. There are, however, some forms of yoga that bring dance into the picture. Shiva Rea does Yoga Trance Dance and some yoga sequences come close to dancing. Classes like Les Mills' BODYBALANCE (previously BodyFlow) or MOSSA's Group Centergy (called Balance and Flex Together at some YMCAs) choreograph yoga movements to music in a way that is certainly approaching dance, although still firmly rooted in fitness. But dancing our yoga might be as simple as practicing to music that speaks to us, building flow into poses and sequences of poses, or simply moving in any way that the music moves us to move our body.

In every yoga class I include an opportunity for some kind of free movement that allows participants to flow at their pace, to move in ways that feel safer than if I called it dance. For instance, a flow that starts with warrior II and alternates between side angle or extended side angle and reverse warrior. (Sometimes called dancing warrior!) After a few cycles, I give people the option to stay with these official yoga postures or create their own shapes and expressions, to embody their warrior spirit—their power and resilience—to create new pathways in the brain and new possibilities in our lives.

Dance involves novel movements and spontaneous freedom to create movement. It rewires the brain and builds new muscle memories. It remaps parts of our bodies that have been neglected or forgotten. Dance is regularly cited as the best antidote to combat dementia and Alzheimer's. We use our brains and our bodies in a rhythm of connection and spontaneity. We don't always know what comes next—in our bodies or in the music or in our minds or our emotions. We can figure it out—or feel it out—as we go along. It can be powerful and empowering to not know what comes next, especially if we find ourselves needing that kind of control.

But getting people to let go enough to move, with or without structure, is often a challenge—even if they are alone, or especially if they are with other people. And yet, moving our bodies with other people is a necessary prerequisite to all kinds of healing. Perhaps the concept of *play* helps to overcome some of the angst? Or maybe the opposite is true—mandated medicine or a work assignment might be the driving force. Ultimately, dance is just movement and not being told how to move can lead to freeze, just as being told how to move can lead to fight or flight or appease.

Movement

Movement means transformation—
Social, cultural, physical—
A promise of a better future
A different way to be

Movement inspires transformation—
Of bodies, ideas, policies
Political and corporal
Shifting sand or muscle

Old wounds may be healed
New wounds may open
And boundaries stretch
Beyond body or mind

We may stumble in our movements
Clashing measures
Failing to measure up
We may repeat the same mistakes

We commit movement to memory
Repeat it
Enough to memorize it
Repeat it enough to forget it was
Memory
And remember
it is perpetual—
Movement.

Move Your Yoga: Choreography

Some people only dance when they are under the influence—which helps to reduce inhibition—or with choreography, which helps to provide a sense of safety. Choreography matches movement to music and can embody the words literally and figuratively; it brings kinesthetic learning to an auditory experience. However, choreography does not necessarily need to be done to music. Moving with the rhythm of the breath in yoga is embodied choreography. Both poetry and choreography can scare some people away. Like poetry, dance is a fine art. While any of us can write poetry and all of us can dance, the art of dance is something altogether different from the booty shake we do while washing dishes or the "dance like no one's watching" that we do behind closed doors or in safer spaces. Choreography resonates as something that requires skills and talents—accessible only to people whose bodies move in certain kinds of ways. But choreography is only another way of communicating—a language of the body, of embodied movement.

I have always loved choreography in fitness classes—learning it, executing it, and before too long, creating my own. Step aerobics is especially fun; there are so many different ways to move around that little box! I have never found success with learning choreography in "real" dance classes; my body just won't do some things and I move slowly. But I haven't really taken many *dance* classes, beyond the tap and ballet of childhood. In Denmark, I joined a dance fitness class that was not the kind of fitness I was used to; it was dance for fitness, not fitness through dance. In junior high, a friend and I took a jazz dance class from an eccentric woman who choreographed the musicals at my parents' church. I remember her teaching us choreography that she was clearly making up on the spot. It kept changing and I felt like it did not fit my body or the music. But who was I to argue with the expert in the room? I could not articulate what felt off about it. After years of creating my own fitness choreography, I understand better. She was not invested, and she was not embodied.

When I create choreography, I create from my body, from my connection to the music, from a solid base of core moves and creative fluctuations. Most of the time, a song speaks to me and suddenly I can't not choreograph it. Sometimes I feel like it choreographs itself. But it has been difficult for me to own my choreography as "real" choreography. It's just fitness, right? I still love it and I most enjoy bringing my choreography into classes, into other people's bodies. Sometimes I am amazed at how much choreography is in my head. It is one thing that I can remember, perhaps because that memory lives in my body as well as my mind.

I was re-inspired to create choreography (and own it!) while participating in a module led by Ananya Chatterjee during the Embodied

Social Justice certificate program that I took with The Embody Lab. What she did in her module was probably pretty out there for many people taking this program. But for me, it was like coming home. Drawing inspiration and wisdom from Alexis Pauline Gumbs's book *Undrowned*, she encouraged us to find our dorsal fins. ("Yes, I need a dorsal fin to navigate all of this transformation"!) I had read *Undrowned* a couple months before and the idea instantly clicked. She encouraged us to "ground in what is needed to activate your dorsal fin, to allow directionality and support from the back side of the body." She explained the ways in which choreography is often about performing. We focus on the front side of the body so that the "interaction becomes about offering or display." She encouraged us to relax ("a lack of straining"), to move about our space. To move backward, to explore. She riffed off of Gumbs's words, asking us to be "grounded and activated from the inside," to find stabilizing practices in these "times of turbulence" so that we can support ourselves and others. Through all of this instruction we were encouraged to just move. The chat was blowing up with questions, concerns, criticisms: but ..., what if ..., I can't.... She addressed each concern with kindness while I wanted to scream—just shut up and move people! Just play with it!

Amidst all of this uncertainty, she stopped and told us that now it was our turn to create our own choreography. I could feel the tension and anxiety in the Zoom room spike at the very moment that my mind/body began to sing, to buzz with excitement. This was my comfort zone. I was reminded just how much choreography intimidates people—how much *movement* scares people. How brave of Ananya to ask us to move in these ways! I was already creating as she attempted to address the angst. She reminded us that choreography is an "embodied way of responding to the world." It is a way of communicating through a series of intentional movements. It doesn't have to be dance. It doesn't have to be anything but movement. Still, the chat blew up with fears and insecurities. For some, the idea got stuck in their heads because their bodies were less mobile, but for many, they were stuck in their heads because of the anxiety that comes with overthinking (even as this anxiety is also felt in the body). I could not help but mourn the lost opportunity for so many people who could not be in their bodies for this practice.

And this mourning turned into my own version of this exercise that I share in "embodied movement" workshops and with the students in my Embodied Social Justice class. We move and discover our dorsal fins, and then I share the choreography that I created and encourage them to do the same. No music, just movement—rhythm and breath. Movement meets us where we are.

As much as I preach freedom through dance, for a long time I stayed in the fitness, and then the fitness dance box. I evolved into offering structure with a taste of freedom. I further evolved when I started teaching (guiding, facilitating) JourneyDance, which is guided movement that I would have been afraid of when I was younger. Yoga movement and choreographed fitness felt much safer. But I've discovered a passion for JourneyDance, as a participant and as a facilitator. In JourneyDance we can move authentically and every dance is different, even when the music is the same. Facilitating JourneyDance is not just about encouraging freedom. It is curating and guiding an experience. It is a different kind of choreography that requires a grounded authenticity. It is holding a space of inspiration and transformation. I am not on a stage or a pedestal. I am on the journey with the participants. We move together while I hold the space and shape the practice and the process.

Bodies on Edge

we feel it
the rise, the beat—
uncontrollable.
in the car, at the store, on the couch
it moves us

we shake: anticipation

we feel it
the rise, the beat—
uncontainable.
inside/outside (beyond reach)
it moves us

we shake: exhilaration

we are bodies on edge;
we are ripe craving movement

sharing space,
our bodies vibrate as one

rising, beating
shaking
   a groove
   a moment
   a lifetime
we feel it
the rise, the beat—

Move Your Yoga: Flash Mob Style

Yoga does not have to be in a studio or on a mat. It does not have to obey predetermined rules. We can practice anytime, anywhere. I have done yoga in hot tubs, on street corners, in my office, in nature. And, of course, yoga breathing is even easier to practice anywhere.

We may get funny looks when we bring yoga to public spaces or we may find a yoga flash mob forming around us!

Yoga and Dance as Healing Modalities

Ultimately, despite their differences, yoga and dance—and movement more generally, especially movement with mindfulness, breath, and meditation—share the category of healing modalities. Human beings have engaged in movement, dancing, breathing, stretching, singing/chanting/sounding, and combinations of all of these for as long as we have been on this earth! Every culture, every group of people, across time and space have engaged in these rituals, rebellions, and recreational activities and they have engaged in them because they heal and connect people in powerful ways. They are also countering oppression.

When we let ourselves play outside of the box of our strict social proprieties, we connect with our very humanness and our innate capacity to heal ourselves. This is science and magic. I've discovered this power even more strongly in my JourneyDance training and restorative yoga training—guided movement and stillness are two modes that were once a source of fear for me, as they are for so many people. But now they are only healing and I aspire to bring this magic to as many people as I can. The problem is that not everyone wants to heal. The excuses we make for why we can't do yoga, or why we can't dance, are often rooted in fear. I get it. I was there once. We are all there, once. And sometimes we revert back there again. Healing is a non-linear process. It takes time.

Those of us who teach, guide, mentor, coach, counsel, encourage, and promote healing often have an uphill battle. *The Salt Eaters*, a 1980 novel by Toni Cade Bambara, opens with a healer, Minnie Ransom, saying to her patient, Velma Henry: "'Are you sure, sweetheart, that you want to be well?'" (3). Velma, an activist, mother, and wife, has attempted suicide and she is having trouble holding onto herself, let alone the stool she is perched upon. Later, Minnie continues, "'cause wholeness is no trifling matter. A lot of weight when you're well'" (10). Staying well—mentally, physically, emotionally, spiritually—is a challenge even in the best of times and circumstance. Minnie Ransom is full of insight and wisdom, noting that some people just aren't ready to "'take away the miseries,'" because without them, "'you take away some folks' reason for living. Their conversation piece anyway'" (16). Being well requires work, patience, self-compassion, and resources. The struggle is real. But as Minnie reminds us, "'got to give it all up, the pain, the hurt, the anger and make room for lovely things to rush in and fill you full'" (16). There's nothing wrong if we "'want to stomp around a little more in the mud puddle … like a little kid … Nothing wrong with that'" (16). We're all just stomping around in the mud, and there's nothing wrong with that. But when we can harness our play toward healing, rather than toward distraction or avoidance, the possibilities abound. When we move, we are moved.

Move (and Be Moved)

When I dance
I find every limitation
of my body
the tight spots
incomplete range of motion
carving old boundaries
around resistant bones
shifting sinew
bracketing an asterisk

When I dance
I find every freedom
of my body
novel movements—
new pathways remolding
the brain
crafting new possibilities
in the body
unbracketing

When I dance
I skirt edges,
scale mountains
expose roots
spin stories
lose myself
in and out of choreography
phrase and rephrase

When I dance
I balance air, clear cobwebs
feet become roots
wrists become wings
body becomes
unwound and remixed
mind becomes landscape
I am moved

Move Your Yoga: Janelle Monáe, "Yoga" (dance "routine")

When my yoga participants are open to it, I include a song with choreographed movements like Lorde's "Glory and Gore" for a Woman Warriors workshop or Janelle Monáe's "Yoga" to get people to let loose and not take themselves, or yoga, so seriously. Monáe's song critiques yoga but also celebrates the freedom of yoga as well as the freedom of "the booty." This is a freedom of physical movement bolstered by women's empowered spaces.

My poem for Janelle Monáe was inspired by my attendance at a Yoga Journal LIVE! conference in New York City; it was a coping mechanism to quell my constant feelings of being a misfit in that space. It is an ode to more than Monáe, to more than yoga.

Let Your Booty Do That Yoga
(For Janelle Monáe)

Tight booties abound
Making breathing impossible,
Making eyes closed undesirable.

I should be focused—
Transcending the body
Expanding the mind
Within myself, beyond limitations

But yoga pants are a practice in distraction.

It's not the one;
It's the many—
The myriad prints and fabrics
Shapes and sizes,
The many moving

> As one synchronous mass
> Of beauty in motion.
>
> Not objects to be ogled
> But subjects to be moved
> Beyond, within, behind
> Centered and expansive—
> The booty taking up as much space as our imaginations.
>
> The mind/body/spirit of our collective power—
> A movement toward transformation.
> Women rock yoga pants like we rock the world.

I had never seen so many colorful, wild versions of yoga pants. And I had never been surrounded by so many beautiful women sporting those yoga pants. It was exhilarating and debilitating. If I can't be the beauty, I can at least admire it when it threatens to drown my sense of self and fledgling confidence! The next year, my mom bought me a pair of what I call my "New York yoga pants." It took a lot of looking and unsuccessful tries to find a pair that fit me. When I wear them I channel Janelle Monáe and let my booty do that yoga! And with sugar skulls and a dramatic design on one leg, they always get a comment, a "like," and a question of where I got them. I only tell part of the story.

*

For this piece of yoga play, we basically just need to do what Janelle Monáe's words tell us to do. Here's a guide:

Play the song

Stand in a wide straddle stretch. (Feet parallel to the sides of your yoga mat, knees a little bit bent, distance comfortable and stable.) You don't have to have a very wide stance!

Inhale and exhale flowing side stretches, reaching and moving with the music.

When the beat picks up, take your movement to a loose upper body pulse. (Arms loose by the sides, bounce the chest and shoulders, squeeze the shoulder blades, lift and drop the ribcage. Bend the knees a bit and move as it feels good to you.)

When they tell you to, lengthen the spine (with knees slightly bent) and hinge forward into a standing straddle stretch. (Hands can rest on the quadriceps, a block, a chair, or the floor.)

When they tell you, let go. Bend your knees, shake your booty. (No one's watching!)

Slowly lift up with a flat back (or round through the spine with hands on the quadriceps for support if that is more comfortable). And then repeat for each of the next two sections of the song. You can even vary the movements in the verse and match movements to the lyrics ... or not!

I'm always a little nervous when I add this song to class. People usually play along. Some people hate it and ignore my instruction. Some people love and embrace it. I was surprised by how many of my nursing students enjoyed this activity. Several commented on how nice it was to break out of the box of yoga and dance. At the very least, it is something a little different and an opportunity to feel, to move, to have fun—to play!

Mindfulness Coloring, "Gush Art," and Zentangling

Yoga can help us recognize and release, but we need other tools as well. It is not difficult to find a wide variety of mindfulness coloring books, for adults and for children. Some are even yoga themed with mandalas, for instance. Others include patterns, animals, nature scenes, or girl power slogans! These resources give us structure and choice within these structures.

When I was working through Jamie Marich's book, *Process Not Perfection*, I was introduced to the concept of gush art, "a term used in expressive arts therapy to suggest uncensored creation with art" (119). I had been doing mindful coloring for a few years; I needed the structure that coloring books provided. But I had started to color without the lines, tentatively reaching toward freedom and self-discovery. In one exercise she asked us to do a coloring page activity, followed by a gush art activity and then to compare the two. I realized that I no longer needed—or wanted—the lines.

Gush art is exactly what it sounds like—no rules, start with an idea (or no idea!) and let it out on the page however it comes out. We may feel a new-found sense of freedom in the permission to create "art" as expression-focused, to be focused on the process rather than the product. It doesn't have to be good.

Gush art is also permission to spill unspent, pent up emotions onto a page rather than onto a person (or the self!), to let the feelings out rather than allow them to spin and do damage from the inside out. While I sometimes think of gush art as being something that is out of control—a result of letting go on the page—it isn't necessarily messy. We might use yoga as a prompt and gush a tree or a mountain, for instance, or our favorite animal pose represented on paper. We can play with the colors that represent each of the chakras or draw circles or spirals or infinity symbols. We might also use art to explore ideas. Certain phrases resonate with me more after I draw them. I'll often start by drawing words and then see what shapes emerge around them.

One of my students introduced me to the Zentangle Method, which provides some structure through framing and instruction. This method is meant to be relaxing and meditative, helping us to increase our awareness, expand our imaginations, and trust our creativity, among other things. ("About the Zentangle Method") Despite the container that Zentangling instructions provide, the results are unique to each individual. Even when the components seem simple—lines, dots, circles, curves—beautiful designs can emerge. As my student reminded us throughout her instruction for a class activity, there are no mistakes.

*

Ultimately, whatever the medium—paper and pen, colored pencils, chalk, collage, paint, clay, or the body itself—play is about letting go. When we let go, play is the very purpose of our movements. We can let go of our focus on the end goal. We can stop counting calories or steps. We can be in the moment and need nothing more. We often admire children's capacity for play, but we also know that children learn about themselves and the world through play. I was a rather serious child; I have had to re-learn how to play. I am still learning. And that is part of the beauty of being open to learning about ourselves and the world—we are never too old to play.

Yoga for Kids of All Ages

I do not have kids and I do not spend a lot of time with kids, but I have taken a couple of trainings that focus on yoga for kids and yoga for childhood trauma. I was not excited about a required training that focused on kids, but it was a lot more fun and informative than I expected it to be! It was different than most of the trainings that I have taken. It was delivered as a set of games that we played, which was then supplemented by information, as opposed to receiving information, which is then supplemented by practicing poses. But the best lesson that I learned from this training is that we all need more play in our lives. Taking yoga outside of the box is not only a way to bring it to kids; it is also a way to get us stodgy adults out of our comfort zones and make us smile and laugh while we are doing yoga.

There are tons of benefits for kids when we bring them yoga—in our schools, in our homes, in our daycare centers. Anywhere! Some of these benefits are obvious: yoga calms the nervous system and can help teach kids to manage their emotions. Yoga builds new pathways in the brain which certainly help a growing brain develop. Yoga provides access to mind/body connections and can help kids feel successful in their bodies. For all of these reasons, and more, yoga is increasingly being put to use in schools—as an opportunity for movement to break up the long days of sitting, as a substitution for traditional detention, and as a means of developing better skills of concentration and coordination. The last few years I have presented at a Zoom conference for Maine teachers, giving them tools for self-care as well as for classroom activities. I hope the few hundred people who have attended my sessions are utilizing both.

When I started making fitness videos for my YMCA (when Covid sent us all into our homes and the Y was providing daycare for essential workers and needed some new activities to do with the kids), I agreed to make a video for kids yoga that the Y would post on its virtual fitness page. I was a little bit nervous about this, especially since my last attempt to provide yoga to kids was pretty disastrous. Half the kids somewhat paid attention to me while the rest ran around like wild animals—and that was for a martial arts class! That was, however, before I was trained. Still.

I came up with a routine that I planned to deliver in an empty room, directed toward a camera and parents who wanted to do yoga at home with their kids. About five minutes before I arrived at the YMCA I found out that I would actually be teaching to real live kids. I tapped into my yoga breaths to calm myself. Did I mention that I don't spend a lot of time with kids? I soon found out that I would be delivering yoga to two different age groups. Keep breathing!

When the first group of kids arrived, they were pretty unruly. They were small—five to six years old, I think. I was shocked how they were instantly engaged and that I kept their attention for the entire 25 minutes! Many of them wanted to be all up in my face. (I tried to breathe less.) They loved laying on the floor and didn't want to get back up. I was shocked with how well it went—yoga is magical!

When the second group arrived, they were old enough to be vocal about how much they did not want to do yoga (eight years old, maybe?). They looked at me skeptically; some said they weren't going to do it and were told they could just sit quietly and watch. Most of their teachers, who were young people in their 20s, didn't take part in the activity, which was not cool. If and when I teach yoga to kids in the future, I will require the teachers to participate as well. We can at least model participation for our kids! The teachers with the first group were willing. I was panicking that the games I had played with the first group would not go well with this group. But again, yoga worked its magic. The kids were instantly involved in the activities and they all participated. When it was over they asked if they could do yoga again!

I do not credit these successes to my skills or my ability to connect with kids—it was mostly the yoga! It is fun and it is something different, but I think that it is also something that can immediately make a difference in how a kid feels—mentally and physically. Other teachers' experiences and research support this claim. There are plenty of online resources to bring yoga to kids. Parents and teachers can immediately take the activities and techniques into their homes and classrooms. We really don't need much—the kids do most of the work for us! When doing yoga with kids, there is no need to hold shapes very long and no need to get hung up on the "right" way of doing something. It's just play! Teaching kids breathing techniques, guiding them through making shapes and expressing ideas through their bodies are powerful tools to teach young people emotional self-regulation and embodiment. We can tell stories and use our imaginations. We can also let go of competition and foster community through collaboration.

To get started, here's a few things to try:

- Start with some breathing. In through the nose out through the nose. Add movement—inhale arms up, exhale arms down. Or break out of the box and move the arms anywhere as they match the inhale (reach away) and exhale (return to center).
- Make some noise with "ocean breath" or, better yet, "Darth Vader" breath. Seriously, what kid doesn't like that one?
- "Horse lips" is a fun one: inhale in through the nose and out through the mouth with loose lips. Kind of like a fart sound, but if we suggest that, we might lose them in that exercise for the rest of the class. This breath technique is a neural reset and is used when working with children on the Autism spectrum, though it is effective for anyone of any age. (Hint: the face has to be relaxed; a trick is to put your fingers on your face below the check bones.)
- Do some down dogs or cat/cow stretches. Encourage moos and meows and waggling tails. They might walk their dog all around the room or flip it into a walking crab.
- Put on some surfing music and ride the waves in warrior II pose. If they have yoga mats—the mat is the surfboard.
- Warriors: do some warrior poses and ask the kids who their favorite warriors are or what the qualities of a warrior are. Ask them to demonstrate these qualities in their poses.
- Balancing tree pose: as we balance, we can ask kids to make the shape of their favorite tree. This can also be done as seed to tree, having the kids start tucked into a "seed" (child's pose) and then water them (or sprinkle fairy dust) and let them grow into the tree.

- Move and freeze. Green light/red light or some other image can work here. Have the kids move around and then freeze into a certain pose or a pose of their choice or just a shape.
- Field of flowers: stand with feet hip width apart, knees slightly bent, hips forward, and twist, gently swinging the arms side to side like we are standing in a field and swaying in the breeze. (I do this in almost every yoga class. My participants call it "the Sarah.")
- Ask kids to invent their favorite superhero pose. Or to make up a pose. They can be quite inventive. We can also have them spell out words by making letter poses. (The kids at the Y went straight to spelling YMCA.)
- Final relaxation (corpse pose). It was surprising to me how much the kids enjoyed lying down quietly on the floor. They actually did not want to get back up! I added Bee's Breath here: inhale through the nose and then exhale with the mouth closed adding a hum. Invite the kids to close their eyes and cover their ears to make the buzzing of the bees even louder.

Again, even though I have outlined yoga for kids here, adults can have just as much fun with these yoga activities—with or without kids! In fact, these are playful ways to reconnect with our inner child, to find the fun and freedom that comes with yoga and life. We could all use a little bit more fun and freedom!

Fearless Fucking Feminists

Now that we have gotten in touch with our inner child, let's come back around to the real world of serious adult subject matter. Feminists are stereotyped as being humorless, and women are stereotyped as being not funny. But being playful in all of our spheres is one key to living fully in our mind/body/spirit and there is always room for humor in yoga. I love to crack yoga jokes, which are the equivalent of dad jokes. They are really only good as embedded in the practice. For instance, as I offer a variety of options, I remind people to breathe, and then I remind them that breathing is not one of the options. Sometimes people laugh. The classic yoga joke is deadpan telling the class that there is no smiling or laughing out loud because yoga is serious business and no fun at all. This is, of course, followed by laughter and a smile, just in case anyone thought that I was serious (and because at least I crack myself up).

I include these last few poems because my (adult, "non-traditional") students love the first two. I mean, who doesn't love a good f-bomb! They are an example of how we can play with feminism, and the second poem, "The (Other) F word," is just as applicable to yoga as a part of the mainstream world of fitness. Both of these poems appeared in my book *Women and Fitness in American Culture*, a book that is pretty much only read by my students in my American Fitness: Culture, Community, and Transformation class. (My students thought the title of my book should have been *Fearless Fucking Feminists*. If only I could be so bold!) Susan Raffo writes: "I like to call anatomy poetry rather than fact; it *evokes something* that then helps us to understand what we are experiencing" (39; my emphasis). Beautiful. This is my hope—to evoke something that helps us to understand what we are experiencing when we practice yoga.

The F Word

Designated by "F"
(as if we did not know the whole word)
Feminist and Fuck
are both *bad words*

You should not call yourself a _____
(and whether a feminist or not)
You should not want to _____

You should not hold political opinions or
Flesh and blood desires

You should not build community or
Break down barriers
between body and mind

You should not ostracize yourself by
qualifying yourself for a label (SLUT)
Pursuing carnal knowledge or
social justice

You should not remember that
Feminists come in a variety of shades

> And fuck is also a four-letter word
> Used for power and to dis-empower
> through many incarnations
>
> F words are flesh—body & soul
> Full of pleasure and passion
> Tools for
> Fearless
> Fucking feminists.

My students often see me as fearless and all I can do is try to live up to their expectations. They are the ones I most often consider to be fearless. For many years, my work teaching fitness classes slowly chipped away at my fears, giving me confidence and agency. In these ways, fitness is also an F word.

The (Other) F Word

> There's the obvious—
> the one among the four letters.
> The other is the one
> that requires its own field
> of interpretation.
> The first is employed for effect—
> anger, frustration, cool.
> The other's avoided
> because of its implications
> or embraced
> for its possibilities.
>
> And then there's fitness—
> an under-the-radar
> F word—
> a tool of patriarchy
> white supremacy
> offering superficial gains
> (flat abs, tight ass)
> rather than embodied transformation.
>
> Bandied about as a means
> for "better bodies"/
> shucked
> for its unattainable image
>
> Fitness as F word is:
> Ripe for reclaiming
> a tool toward empowerment,
> critical perspective,
> transformation.

> A way of life—
> of balance and flexibility,
> strength and endurance,
> inspiration and energy.
>
> Connections between
> body and mind
> self and community.
>
> Employed for effect
> avoided or embraced
> Fitness
> enhances each of the other important
> F words
> in myriad ways.

I have moved away from fitness, in favor of conscious, embodied movement. This last poem was inspired by writing *Demystifying American Yoga*, thinking about the qualities of yoga that make it a kind of curse word for some people. It speaks to the themes and arguments I make about yoga, riffing off of the same theme of charged and forbidden language. If yoga is only a workout or is viewed as something that conflicts with Christian beliefs, then it is in conflict with the essence of yoga. This poem also speaks to the ways in which yoga is misunderstood, used, and abused as well as the ways in which it can transcend any mis-use. If we let yoga be defined by the systems and structures that shape and contain all of us, then we are letting yoga be limited by our fears of scarcity and our perceptions of a lack of control over our own bodies and minds.

Yoga Is a 4-Letter Word

> some are drawn to it
> like moths to light
> others turn away
> out of fear
> or disgust
> or disinterest
> or ignorance
>
> Yoga is a 4-letter word
>
> when white women speak it
> they better bow to tradition
> or bring something
> to back it up

when not-white women speak it
the gatekeepers close ranks or
lift them up onto pedestals
both still
something less than human

when men speak it
authority ensues
assumes guru status
and some take advantage of
the power they
hold teach inspire mold
and some take advantage of
the bodies
that surrender in their wake
groping
for something more

when capitalism speaks it
dollars signs light
their eyes
greed grasps for authenticity
tramples possibilities
cuts ties that bind
lineages cracking open
union and
the interconnectedness
of all things not able
to be bought and sold

Yoga is a 4-letter word

and yet,
when we speak the language
of yoga with our
bodies/minds/hearts/spirits
in communities and cauldrons
of healing, growing, loving—
practicing—
we transcend the limitations
of language turning
power-over structures into
embodied
empowered
connected
grounded unbound and expansive love…

Love is a 4-letter word
At the center
Of yoga's world(s)

Play as Self-Study: The Remix

Every time I take a new training, read a new book, watch a video, or take someone else's class, I engage in self-study and the art of play. We have to try new things to grow and we have to try new yoga things to grow as yoga teachers, students, and practitioners. We can always come back to our favorite things, but if we don't play around in the yoga mud, we might just lose our passion for it. For instance, I know from experience that hot yoga is not the yoga for me and I was surprised at how much I fell in love with restorative yoga. Now I want all my yoga to at least have a restorative element.

I am grateful to the many teachers that I have had who teach me not only about yoga, but also about myself. It's impossible for me to remember every yoga teacher and trainer I have had. As I mentioned before, my formal 200-hour training spanned across 13 years and I never really expected to go anywhere with it, let alone continue my training past these 200 hours, let alone to write a book about yoga. But here I am, close to an additional 300 hours of training and playing with yoga in one of the modes I most enjoy—writing. So here's a short shout out to the teachers who have resonated most with me over the years:

Bo Forbes cracked my yoga world open with a "Yoga for Empaths" workshop in 2015. Not only did I change my approach to yoga, but I also changed my approach to my life. I have taken a number of different on-line and in-person trainings with her and have read her book, *Yoga for Emotional Balance,* and some of her blogs and occasional social media posts. I appreciate her blend of neuroscience and practical tools for taking care of ourselves. I also appreciate how she is unapologetically herself. This is, at least for me, one of the most important qualities in a yoga teacher.

While there is much to learn about yoga via social media, I rarely spend time in these spaces and, thus, can credit almost none of my yoga journey to online resources. I don't have a habit of listening to podcasts or scrolling through Instagram; I appreciate these resources, but I'm busy and old school. People sometimes send me links and posts, but I rarely go looking for them. Most of my teachers have been teachers to me only through their books. I love books.

I have too many books, if that is possible. (I don't think it is.) Despite my bread and butter job as a professor (a scholar, though I have trouble embracing this designation of my work), most scholarly resources mostly bore me. They are so often so far removed from the embodied, felt experience that drives my transdisciplinary work. They are playing the game of scholarship, research, and publication, and they are important. But I often find them to be dry and long-winded. I write for an audience that is outside of academia, but not far removed. These are the kinds of books I like to read, the kinds of books I cite in my work, and the kinds of books written by, for instance, Gail Parker, who is absolutely brilliant and accessible. My students and I enjoy her books and her insights that focus on race-based trauma but speak to the universality of both trauma and yoga and our experiences of healing and transformation. I found Gail Parker after finding Michelle Cassandra Johnson, whose book was the first book I chose for the class I teach to nursing students. And *Yoke* is a favorite, though I don't follow Jessamyn Stanley more than sporadically. I found Nityda Gessel soon after, and Zahabiyah A. Yamasaki via Gessel a few years later. After sending this book off for publication, one of my next projects is to dig into their self-paced trauma-informed teaching trainings (which I purchased as a package deal). There is always more to learn. And I have learned so much from Susan Raffo's *Liberated to the Bone*, which I read in the last stretch of my writing. She cemented many of my examples (and has so much more to offer!).

Outside of reading books, and a few conferences, most of my yoga training (nearing 500 hours) has been through YogaFit. In YogaFit, Skila Ramirez, Kristen Mabry, Kristy Manuel, Kelly Holloman Gardner, Katie Shuver, Shaye Molendyke, Alison Presley, and Sandi Call were some of the best teachers I have had in any educational setting. While I have had a couple of trainers who were not impressive, these were few and far between. There are so many amazing women who are trainers and teachers for YogaFit; they make this yoga school what it is and continue to grow and expand the programs far beyond Beth Shaw's original vision of YogaFit as yoga that could be taught in health clubs. The team that she has assembled to grow her vision is phenomenal. One thing that I love the most about YogaFit is that they focus on how to teach yoga and how to make yoga accessible to "every body."

They have greatly expanded their trauma-informed offerings and have a training on almost every aspect of yoga imaginable. The women who train instructors have very full lives outside of YogaFit, with an impressive range of "real jobs" that are sometimes related to yoga and sometimes not. They are passionate, accessible, and knowledgeable. Almost all of them are white women. I value their teaching and positive, transformative community impact, locally and beyond.

The only thing that I have found lacking in YogaFit trainings is a social justice and critical consciousness approach. I filter everything through my critical lens and supplement what I learn with feminist and queer resources. So far, I have mostly found social justice connections in books, articles, listserves, and some local connections. (I live and work in Maine and we are generally ten to twenty years behind all trends!) The intersections of yoga, embodied movement, and conscious dance with somatics and social and cultural theory and practice is where most of my connections to yoga and social justice are found, as well as through reading and practice. I share the wisdom of all of these works here, in *Demystifying American Yoga*, in this context of reimagining American yoga. This is the place where my life's work has brought me—embodied social justice—and I plan to continue to explore this ground and bring more insights to my students, my community, and to my own healing journey.

Learning is circular—ideas, concepts, inspirations, and approaches ebb and flow, stick and fade. We have to regularly remind ourselves of things that we already know and/or learn them in a new way. And then, sometimes a particular issue with our body/mind or mind/body/spirit arises and we are led toward—or dropped in the middle of—a realm we didn't expect. Trauma brought me deeper into yoga. Healing brought me to JourneyDance. These embodied movements are powerful, magical, transformative. Transformation is always in process. Self-study is a form of play that we can use as we continue our life-long practice and journey with—and beyond—yoga. What's your next step?

*

As we conclude our practice (to be continued, always), we begin to transition from whatever position we have chosen for our final relaxation. We might give ourselves permission to stay right where we are for as long as we like. We might begin to find micro movements in our hands, fingers, wrists, toes, feet, and ankles. We might wiggle our legs, knees, and hips, ribcage, back, chest, and shoulders. We might press the back of our head into the floor and gently roll it from side to side. We might reach overhead, stretching and yawning, like we are just waking up.

We might bring one foot at a time to the earth, rocking our knees side to side, massaging the low back/sacrum, letting this movement guide us onto one side, supporting the head and neck with an arm or any props we choose. We might tuck ourselves into a seed, preparing for new growth, recognizing, as Gail Parker reminds us: "A seed holds within it the potential to become what it is. It cannot be anything else" (88). We are the power and potential of this seed.

As we push ourselves up to a seated position, we find our sits bones on the earth beneath us. We might sway, shift, move our head and neck gently and lengthen our spine. Perhaps we inhale and gather up all of the positive energy we have created for ourselves and for each other. And as we exhale, we let this wash down the front side of our bodies to heart center.

Perhaps we press our hands together or leave a little space between them or layer our hands over heart center, letting the next inhale bring in love and compassion for ourselves through heart center, and letting the next exhale move love and compassion out into the room around us, and beyond us.

At the end of each practice, we find ourselves renewed, rejuvenated, resourced, and ready to face what comes next. Here, at this intersection, the essence and light in me greets the essence and light in you.

Namaste.

Conclusions

Throughout *Demystifying American Yoga*, I have played with an American tone and attitude that is meant to antagonize in ways that are less gentle than my pedagogical practices in the academic classrooms and community spaces where I do my daily work. This American tone is a persona that is both me and not me at the same time. It is a tone that embodies American idealism (and perhaps exceptionalism) in ways that are both purposeful and unconscious. It is a tone that I hope reflects back to the reader the problems and promises of American yoga. I have aimed to model curiosity and authenticity—to invite readers into internal and external explorations of ourselves and this thing called yoga. I have aimed to demystify and to reimagine what yoga is and what it can be, but ultimately, this is a collective process.

Jivana Heyman argues that if it's not *yoga*, it's simply *embodied movement*. He cautions us about which word we choose to use to describe our offerings: "The challenge here is how your practice can be both creative and traditional. It means that if I'm teaching or practicing yoga, and using the word yoga instead of *embodied movement*, then I'm connecting to an ancient lineage of spiritual seekers who were dedicated to traveling on an inward journey to discover the truth of who they are" (173). From where we stand today, the long lineage of yoga is not a straight path. It meanders and borrows from traditions that parallel or intersect with yoga. There are multiple origin points, innovations, conglomerations, appropriations, divergences, and possibilities, even before yoga was introduced to U.S. audiences. There are many different spiritual seekers, ancient and contemporary. So what exactly is *American yoga* and what can it be?

The picture of American yoga that we see is all surfaces—trends, bendable bodies, products, representations, and appropriation. What we experience is sometimes this version, but it can also be something deeper, more meaningful, more transformative. American yoga is most certainly the surface and glitter, the commodified and marketed, the fitness and sport, the exclusionary and elitist—everything that creates a mainstream, institutionalized, exploitative enterprise. But this is one of America's faces, and if we let this be the face of our yoga, then we are leaving out what are, perhaps, the most powerful parts of our yoga and our country—the marginalized, feminist, queer, grassroots, underground, interconnected, creative, innovative, embodied, and exploratory elements that engage so many of us. When we focus on the surface, we are ignoring the healing and transformative power that cannot be contained or commodified by mainstream America. We are playing the game of power.

Resmaa Menakem offers "body and breath practices" that provide "connections with other bodies—in groups, neighborhoods, and communities" (132). Most of the practices he offers "are ancient" (140) and intuitive, part of many religions, and practiced by slaves on plantations (141), as well as having the backing of scientific research. These practices are long traditions and contemporary tools; some of them are *yoga*, even though he rarely uses this word. He notes the practices are familiar because "They are family and communal strategies that African Americans have used for generations ... to survive, remain resilient, settle our bodies, and alleviate trauma for hundreds of years" (191). These *embodied practices* are a "shared history" (191). What he is describing are *embodied movements* utilized in waves of social and cultural movement as well as for survival, connection, growth, and transformation. Ultimately, what Menakem offers is *American* yoga—American applications of *embodied movement*.

*

I continue to try to wrap my head around all of the arguments that shape our understanding and practice. If we argue that there is something unique to American yoga that needs to be explored, exploded, unpacked, reimagined, and tapped toward individual and collective transformation, is this not simply an extension of American exceptionalism? If we argue that embodied movements are ancient and come from diverse origins, and that these diverse origins shape American yoga, are we excusing the cultural appropriation of yoga? If we argue that yoga is a helpful tool for moving trauma out of our bodies, of processing the "dirty pain" that Menakem writes about, of transforming individual bodies as well as the body of our nation, should we really be using the term *embodied movements* instead?

If what we create from yoga—individually and collectively, in the U.S. and beyond—is something other than yoga, then it is kin. Creativity, Heyman argues, is "literally the embodiment of spirituality" (173). We have to create and re-create mind/body/spirit movements to fit the contours of our lives. If American yoga can embody all of the contradictions that come with our current cultural moment, our reckoning, our intergenerational trauma, our fear, our disconnection, our hopes and dreams, it is something other than yoga while it is also fundamentally yoga. Regardless of what we call it, yoga is a universal spirituality in a cultural context (in the U.S. and beyond) that desperately needs embodied practices toward individual and collective healing and transformation. No one can own yoga, but we can all benefit from its power—individually and collectively, now and into the future that we build together.

*

While Embodied Movement is far more accurate to what I offer in my academic and community teaching, this phrase has not yet made its way into popular consciousness. People know what yoga is, even if they only know the superficial cultural representations and don't actually know what the eight-limbed path of yoga is, or if they think yoga is just a bunch of stretching. In my experience (so far!) people do not know what *embodied movement* means and they are, in turn, intimidated and less likely to try an offering with a title like "Embodied Movements for Transformation" than they are a class called "Yoga," even if the content is the same. As a word and concept, embodiment is scary. Movement is vague and, thus, also scary. The word *yoga* has made its way into all kinds of popular spaces. Even so, yoga might be intimidating even if it is a familiar term— or maybe because it is familiar enough to scare people away from their stereotyped assumptions or fear of physical practices (or internal exploration) in public spaces.

If not for the familiarity that *yoga* provides, I might stop using the word right now; I might argue that this book is not actually about yoga at all. I might argue that American yoga is, in fact, simply a commodified, appropriated, capitalistic enterprise with no grey areas. But, at the same time, yoga is a foundation for the embodied movements that I practice and teach. Yoga is a touchstone of my training—the moment when I stopped thinking about fitness and exercise as a practice for only the body. This moment is not a singular point on the timeline of my education, growth, practice, or teaching. It is not a lone star. Yoga is intertwined with the academic ideas about cultural criticism, feminism, and social justice that I have elucidated in the practice of writing *Demystifying American Yoga*. It is part and parcel with my training as a fitness instructor—a teacher of dance, and step aerobics, and all things recognizable as strength training and cardio. Yoga echoes the spiritual and embodied practices that undergird my training as a JourneyDance facilitator and the embodied movement programs that I create and teach, in academic and community spaces. Yoga, more than once, has saved my life. Yoga is a starting point and a place to return to. Yoga is one thing and it is many things. Yoga is a way of connecting to the past, of accessing the present, and of building a better future. Yoga is an ancient tradition and a renewable resource. If I claim to be writing about yoga, teaching yoga, practicing yoga am I claiming something that is not mine to claim? Is it mine to claim only because it is also yours to claim, because it is ours to claim? Is it ours to claim because yoga is ultimately for *every* body?

We should keep asking questions as we practice—as we move our bodies and engage our mind/body/spirit. And maybe we should not get hung up on a word, a label for something that is bigger than we are. Because American Yoga is more than the surface, more than the sum of its parts, more than what can be quantified. It is past, present, and future—a tool, a way of life, a way of relating to ourselves and to others, a way of being in our bodies and in the world. And if we all had a little more yoga in our lives, then quite obviously, the world would be a better place.

EXPAND (Works Cited)

Demystifying American Yoga includes a lot of references; the citations below are divided between works cited and works referenced. I have done my best to fully cite the works I have quoted or paraphrased from. Works mentioned in passing examples (songs, oracle decks) are not included because they can be easily found via your favorite internet search engine (and/or the citation details are mostly inconsequential). In some cases I have chosen not to cite specifics to retain anonymity, and in other cases I do not have a single source to cite because the examples and information I share are from nearly twenty years of accumulated knowledge.

If there is something you cannot find, please feel free to contact me (my contact info is also easy to find!). All of these citations are offered toward further self-study. I also have further resources available via my website www.thespiralgoddesscollective.com.

Works Cited

"About the Zentangle Method." Zentangle, zentangle.com/pages/about-the-zentangle-method.

Alshami, Ali M. "Pain: Is It All in the Brain or the Heart?" *Current Pain and Headache Reports*, vol. 23, no. 12, 14 Nov. 2019, 88, doi:10.1007/s11916-019-0827-4.

Ballard, Jacoby. *A Queer Dharma: Yoga and Meditations for Liberation.* North Atlantic Books, 2021.

Bambara, Toni Cade. *The Salt Eaters.* Random House, 1980.

Barkataki, Susanna. *Embrace Yoga's Roots: Courageous Ways to Deepen Your Practice.* Ignite Yoga & Wellness Institute, 2020.

———. "How to Decolonize Your Yoga Practice." OpenDemocracy, 13 July 2015, www.opendemocracy.net/en/transformation/how-to-decolonize-your-yoga-practice/.

———. "How to Decolonize Your Yoga Practice." Susannabarkataki.com, 25 Sept. 2018, updated 10 Mar. 2020, www.susannabarkataki.com/post/how-to-decolonize-your-yoga-practice.

———. "You're Not Indian Enough—Embodied Story in Practice." Susannabarkataki.com, 11 Aug. 2020, updated 14 Nov. 2020, www.susannabarkataki.com/post/you-re-not-indian-enough-embodied-in-story-in-practice.

"bell hooks: Critical Consciousness for Political Resistance." South End Press Collective. *Talking About a Revolution: Interviews with Michael Albert, Noam Chomsky, Barbara Ehrereich, bell hooks, Peter Kwong, Winona LaDuke, Manning Marable, Urvashi Vaid, and Howard Zinn.* South End Press, 1998, pp. 59–75.

Bondy, Dianne. "The Black History of Yoga: A Short Exploration of Kemetic Yoga." Yoga International, n.d., https://yogainternational.com/article/view/the-black-history-of-yoga/.

Boyson, Elise. "May E-News: Ahimsa & Roe v. Wade, Older Americans Month, Community Events, And More!" Sea Change Yoga. Received by Sarah Hentges, 11 May 2022.

brown, adrienne maree. *Emergent Strategy: Shaping Change, Changing Worlds.* Emergent Strategy Series. AK Press, 2017.

———. *Holding Change: The Way of Emergent Strategy Facilitation and Mediation.* Emergent Strategy Series. AK Press, 2021.

———. *Pleasure Activism: The Politics of Feeling Good.* Emergent Strategy Series. AK Press, 2019.

Brown, Richard P., and Patricia L. Gerbarg. *The Healing Power of the Breath: Simple Techniques to Reduce Stress and Anxiety, Enhance Concentration, and Balance Your Emotions.* Shambhala, 2012.

Chaterjee, Ananya. "Module 13: The Artful Body." Section 2—How Justice Lives in the Body, Embodied Social Justice Certificate, 50 Hour Certificate Program, The Embody Lab, 24 May 2021.

Cooper, Anderson. "Cornel West Celebrates Multiracial Protest Coalition While Warning Against 'Neo-Fascist Clapdown.'" *Newsweek*, 10 June 2020, www.newsweek.com/potify-cooper-cornel-west-george-floyd-funeral-memorial-service-killing-police-black-lives-matter-1509995.

Ehrenreich, Barbara. *Natural Causes: An Epidemic of Wellness, the Certainty of Dying, and Killing Ourselves to Live Longer.* Twelve, 2019.

The Embody Lab. "The Embodiment Sale starts today! SAVE up to 50% on our best-selling collection." Received by Sarah Hentges, 25 Nov. 2021.

Emerson, David, and Elizabeth Hopper. *Overcoming Trauma Through Yoga: Reclaiming Your Body.* North Atlantic Books, 2011.

Evans, Stephanie Y. *Black Women's Yoga History: Memoirs of Inner Peace.* SUNY Press, 2021.

Forbes, Bo. *Yoga for Emotional Balance: Simple Practices to Help Relieve Anxiety and Depression.* Shambhala, 2011.

Gesell, Nityda. *Embodied Self-Awakening: Somatic Practices for Trauma Healing and Spiritual Evolution.* W.W. Norton, 2023

Gumbs, Alexis Pauline. *Undrowned: Black Feminist Lessons from Marine Mammals.* Emergent Strategy Series. AK Press, 2020.

Haines, Staci K. *The Politics of Trauma: Somatics, Healing, and Social Justice.* North Atlantic Books, 2019.

Harris, Nadine Burke. *The Deepest Well: Healing the Long-Term Effects of Childhood Trauma and Adversity.* Mariner Books, 2021.

HeartMath. "Quick Coherence® Technique." HeartMath, Inc., www.heartmath.com/quick-coherence-technique/.

Hentges, Sarah. *Women and Fitness in American Culture.* McFarland, 2013.

Hersey, Tricia. *Rest Is Resistance: A Manifesto.* Little, Brown Spark, 2022.

Heyman, Jivana. *Yoga Revolution: Building a Practice of Courage and Compassion.* Shambhala, 2021.

Hobart, Hi'ilei Julia Kawehipuaakahaopulani, and Tamara Kneese. "Radical Care: Survival Strategies for Uncertain Times." *Social Text*, vol. 38, no. 1 (142), 1 March 2020, 1–16, https://doi.org/10.1215/01642472-7971067.
Hoffman, Dirk. UBNow. "West urges 'love warriors' to lead battle against hatred." UBNow, 4 Mar. 2021, www.buffalo.edu/ubnow/stories/2021/03/west-beyond-knife.html.
hooks, bell. "Theory as Liberatory Practice." *Teaching to Transgress: Education as the Practice of Freedom*. Routledge, 1994, pp. 39–52.
Horton, Carol. *Yoga Ph.D.: Integrating the Life of the Mind and the Wisdom of the Body*. Kleio Books, 2012.
Hotep, Yasir Ra. "What is Kemetic Yoga™?" *Kemetic YogaSkills*, kemeticyogaskills.com/.
Howard, Leslie. *Pelvic Liberation: Using Yoga, Self-Inquiry, and Breath Awareness for Pelvic Health*. Leslie Howard Yoga, 2017.
Johnson, Michelle Cassandra. *Skill in Action: Radicalizing Your Yoga Practice to Create a Just World*. 2017. Shambhala, 2020.
Kim, Jina B., and Sami Schalk. "Reclaiming the Radical Politics of Self-Care: A Crip-of-Color Critique." *The South Atlantic Quarterly*, vol. 20, no. 2, 1 April 2021, 325–342, Duke UP, https://doi.org/10.1215/00382876-8916074.
Kingston, Maxine Hong. *The Woman Warrior: Memoir of a Girlhood Among Ghosts*. Knopf, 1976.
Lasater, Judith Hanson. *Living Your Yoga: Finding the Spiritual in Everyday Life*. 2nd ed., Rodmell Press, 2015.
Law, Naomi. "Celebrate freedom but understand freedom is not free." *Galesburg Register-Mail*, 18 July 2022, www.galesburg.com/story/opinion/columns/2022/07/18/naomi-law-celebrate-freedom-but-understand-freedom-not-free/10011852002/.
Long, Jana, director. *The Uncommon Yogi: A History of Blacks and Yoga in the U.S.* Produced by the Black Yoga Teachers Alliance, YouTube, 2016.
Long, Jana. Foreword. *Black Women's Yoga History: Memoirs of Inner Peace*. SUNY Press, 2021, pp. xi–xiii.
Lorde, Audre. *A Burst of Light*. Firebrand Books, 1988.
Marich, Jamie. *Process Not Perfection: Expressive Arts Solutions for Trauma Recovery*. Creative Mindfulness Media, 2019.
Menakem, Resmaa. *My Grandmother's Hands: Racialized Trauma and the Pathway to Mending Our Hearts and Bodies*. Central Recovery Press, 2017.
National Women's Studies Association. "2022 NWSA Call for Papers." www.drake.edu/media/departmentsoffices/wgs/2022%20NWSA%20Conference%20Call%20for%20Papers.pdf.
———. "Yoga for NWSA Members: Oct. 12–Dec. 21" Received by Sarah Hentges, 9 Oct. 2020.
Orloff, Judith. *Thriving as an Empath: 365 Days of Self-Care for Sensitive People*. Sounds True Adult, 2022.
Parker, Gail. *Restorative Yoga for Ethnic and Race-Based Stress and Trauma*. Singing Dragon, 2020.
———. *Transforming Ethnic and Race-Based Traumatic Stress with Yoga: Rest, Reflect, and Renew*. Singing Dragon, 2021.
Piepzna-Samarasinha, Leah Lakshmi. *Care Work: Dreaming Disability Justice*. Arsenal Pulp Press, 2018.
———. *The Future Is Disabled: Prophecies, Love Notes and Mourning Songs*. Arsenal Pulp Press, 2022.
Raffo, Susan. *Liberated to the Bone: Histories. Bodies. Futures*. Emergent Strategy Series No.7. AK Press, 2022.

Rashid, Taz DJ. "About." *Spotify,* open.spotify.com/artist/2XvQyfssNbXYWcOkKaWYlx.

Redmond, Caroline. "11 of the Fiercest and Bravest Woman Warriors and Female Fighters Throughout History." All That Is Interesting, 7 Nov. 2021, Allthatsinteresting.com/women-warriors

Róisín, Fariha. *Who Is Wellness For? An Examination of Wellness Culture and Who It Leaves Behind.* Harper, 2022.

Schwartz, Arielle. *Therapeutic Yoga for Trauma Recovery: Applying the Principles of Polyvagal Theory for Self-Discovery, Embodied Healing, and Meaningful Change.* PESI Publishing, Inc., 2022.

Sederer, Lloyd I. "What Does 'Rat Park' Teach Us About Addiction?" *Psychiatric Times,* MJH Life Sciences, 10 June 2019, www.psychiatrictimes.com/view/what-does-rat-park-teach-us-about-addiction.

Sol Rising. "About." *Spotify,* open.spotify.com/artist/1BdgyHJZID1ceLLg31KyAv.

"Spiritual bypass." *Wikipedia,* en.wikipedia.org/wiki/Spiritual_bypass.

Stanley, Jessamyn. *Every Body Yoga: Let Go of Fear, Get on the Mat, Love Your Body.* Workman Publishing Group, 2017.

———. *Yoke: A Yoga of My Self-Acceptance.* Workman Publishing Group, 2021.

Tatum, Beverly Daniels. "Defining Racism: Can We Talk?" *Why Are All the Black Kids Sitting Together in the Cafeteria? And Other Conversations About Race.* Revised Edition, Basic Books, 2017, pp. 83–97.

Tawwab, Nedra Glover. *Set Boundaries, Find Peace: A Guide to Reclaiming Yourself.* TarcherPerigee, 2021.

Taylor, Keeanga-Yamahtta Taylor. "The Combahee River Collective Statement." *How We Get Free: Black Feminism and the Combahee River Collective.* Haymarket Books, 2017, pp. 15–27.

Taylor, Sonya Renee. *The Body Is Not an Apology: The Power of Radical Self-Love.* Berrett-Koehler Publishers, 2021.

Tygielski, Shelly. *Sit Down to Rise Up: How Radical Self-Care Can Change the World.* New World Library, 2021.

Weintraub, Amy. *Yoga for Depression: A Compassionate Guide to Relieve Suffering Through Yoga.* Broadway Books, 2004.

Yamasaki, Zahabiyah A. *Trauma-Informed Yoga for Survivors of Sexual Assault: Practices for Healing and Teaching with Compassion.* W.W. Norton, 2022.

"Yoga Sutras of Patanjali." *Wikipedia,* en.wikipedia.org/wiki/Yoga_Sutras_of_Patanjali.

Y12SR. "Y12SR Meetings: Healing in Community." Give Back Yoga Foundation, www.y12sr.com/meetings.

Works Referenced

Arao, Brian, and Kristi Clemens. "From Safe Spaces to Brave Spaces: A New Way to Frame Dialogue Around Diversity and Social Justice." *The Art of Effective Facilitation.* Stylus Publishing, LLC, 2013.

Black Yoga Teachers Alliance, blackyogateachersalliance.org/.

Hentges, Sarah. *Girls on Fire: Transformative Heroines in Young Adult Dystopian Literature.* McFarland, 2018.

Heyman, Jivana. *Accessible Yoga: Poses and Practices for Every Body.* Shambhala, 2019.

hooks, bell. *Feminist Theory: From Margin to Center.* South End Press, 1984.

Horton, Carol, and Roseanne Harvey. *21st Century Yoga: Culture, Politics, and Practice.* Kleio Books, 2012.

Levine, Peter. *Waking the Tiger: Healing Trauma.* North Atlantic Books, 1997.
Maté, MD Gabor. *In the Realm of Hungry Ghosts: Close Encounters with Addiction.* North Atlantic Books, 2010.
Rosen, Tommy. *Recovery 2.0: Move Beyond Addiction and Upgrade Your Life.* Hay House, 2014.
Saradananda, Swami. *Mudras for Modern Life: Boost Your Health, Re-Energize Your Life, Enhance Your Yoga and Deepen Your Meditation.* Watkins Publishing, 2015.
Swanson, Ann. *Science of Yoga: Understand the Anatomy and Physiology to Perfect Your Practice.* DK, 2019.
van der Kolk, Bessel. *The Body Keeps the Score: Brain, Mind, and Body in the Healing of Trauma.* Penguin, 2015.
Weiss, Robert. *Prodependence: Beyond the Myth of Codependency.* Health Communications, 2022.
Wong, Alice. *Disability Visibility: First-Person Stories from the Twenty-First Century.* Vintage Books, 2020.
Yamasaki, Zahabiyah A., and Evelyn Rosario Andry. *Trauma-Informed Yoga Affirmation Card Deck.* W.W. Norton, 2022.

Index

AA (Alcoholics Anonymous) 106
ableism 17, 118, 143; *see also* disability
academia 10, 14, 21, 42, 56, 63, 69, 74, 86, 99, 109, 119, 125, 128, 142, 163, 165–67, 168, 169, 207–8, 233, 235, 236; *see also* interdisciplinary; teaching; women's studies
Accessible Yoga 42, 120, 240; *see also* Heyman, Jivana
ACEs (Adverse Childhood Experiences) 112
activism 31, 87, 109, 187; *see also* social justice
addiction 37, 105–9, 240
ADHD (Attention-Deficit Hyperactivity Disorder) 45
Africa xii, 7, 61, 64, 89, 95, 171
African American 169, 170, 234; history 171; studies 83
aging 71, 86, 119
Alexander, Dr. Bruce 106
Alshami, Ali M. 27, 237
American 8, 14, 16–18, 31, 35–6, 40, 43–44, 47, 49–50, 51–2, 57, 69, 89, 92, 94, 122, 137, 168, 175, 180, 186–87, 188, 196, 204, 233; culture 6, 36, 37, 38, 45, 71, 72, 82, 85, 92, 97, 105, 112, 114, 115, 119, 123, 124, 132, 150–51, 155, 161, 162, 180, 191, 195, 200; exceptionalism 10, 150, 233, 234; mainstream 12, 37, 41, 42, 85, 92–93, 117, 118, 119, 122, 128, 155, 162, 164, 179, 188, 234; studies 9, 69, 83; revolution 4, 10
American yoga 3, 4, 5, 6, 8, 9, 10–11, 13, 14, 39, 42–43, 50, 69, 72, 86, 91, 92–93, 95, 100, 115, 118, 122, 123, 137, 139, 147, 168–69, 171, 173, 176, 196, 201, 231, 233–36; *see also* yoga
anatomy 45–46, 182, 225
Anderson Cooper 360 147, 238
anxiety 21, 23, 24, 35, 37, 45, 55, 59, 62, 81, 158, 213; *see also* depression; mental health
Arao and Clemens 109, 240
art 47, 54, 62, 63, 76, 104, 109, 135, 136, 141, 145, 153, 174, 193, 200, 207, 212, 219–20
asana 19, 38, 94, 96, 120, 123, 188; *see also* yoga

Bad Feminist 162; *see also* Gay, Roxane
balance 27, 28, 43, 44, 53, 71, 73, 81–82, 108, 133, 141, 160, 163, 182, 198, 201–2, 223, 227; imbalance 81, 95; life balance 57, 81–82, 104, 107, 162, 180, 190, 195, 198
Ballard, Jacoby 15, 40, 69, 73–74, 83–5, 87, 93, 108–9, 115–17, 180, 184, 196–98, 237; *see also* A Queer Dharma
Bambara, Toni Cade 216, 237; *see also The Salt Eaters*
Barkataki, Susanna 15, 34, 39–40, 87, 91–99, 184, 196, 237; *see also Embrace Yoga's Roots*
Betts, Reginald Dwayne 208; *see also Felon*
binaries 38, 81–2
BIPOC (Black, Indigenous & People of Color) 12–13, 34, 52, 90, 92–95, 99, 112, 120, 122, 161, 190; "The Black History of Yoga" 94, 238
Black feminism *see* feminism
Black Feminist Thought 170; *see also* Collins, Patricia Hill
Black Lives Matter 14
Black Women's Yoga History 170–71, 238–39; *see also* Evans, Stephanie Y.
The Body Is Not an Apology 127, 240; *see also* Taylor, Sonya Renee
Boggs, Grace Lee 172–73
Bondy, Dianne 73, 91, 94–5, 120, 238; *see also Yoga for Everyone*

243

boundaries 38, 125, 129, 149–50, 164, 173, 192; conceptual 30, 117, 199, 203, 211, 216; geographical 4, 8, 94
Boyson, Elise ix-x, 189–90, 238; *see also* Sea Change Yoga
breath 9, 13–15, 20–28, 33, 35, 38, 44, 55–56, 58, 67, 75, 81, 82, 103, 108, 124, 141, 144, 156, 158, 159, 178, 185, 198, 209, 211, 214, 215, 223, 224, 234, 238, 239; conscious breathing 21, 22, 47, 142, 161, 169; *see also* pranayama
British 39, 40, 91, 94, 95
brown, adrienne maree vi, 17, 145, 171–74, 185, 238; *see also Emergent Strategy*; *Holding Change*; *Pleasure Activism*
Brown and Gerbarg 24, 144, 238; *see also The Healing Power of the Breath*
Buddhism 15, 179–80, 197
A Burst of Light 124, 239; *see also* Lorde, Audre
Butler, Octavia 34–5, 148, 156, 172, 174
BYTA (Black Yoga Teachers Alliance) 170, 239, 240

capitalism 2, 10, 52, 70, 88, 108, 128, 148, 162, 173, 187, 228
care 52, 58, 63, 92, 104, 112–13, 119–20, 121, 125, 127, 128, 132, 147, 175, 176, 186–87, 191; caregivers 113; collective care 117, 127, 128, 142, 191; radical care 127, 239; *see also* self-care
Care Work 119, 239; *see also* Piepzna-Samarasinha, Leah Lakshmi
chakras 26, 36, 56, 61, 138, 153–155, 220
change 4, 14, 34–5, 39, 41, 44, 49, 55, 56, 61, 67, 82, 86, 96, 109, 111, 112, 114, 119, 127, 128, 133, 148, 154, 156–57, 162, 163, 172, 176, 184–85, 195, 196, 200, 202, 203, 229, 238, 240; climate 111; collective 194; political 129; social 40, 97; *see also* transformation
Chatterjee, Ananya 212–13; *see also* The Embody Lab
Choudhury, Bikram 79
Christianity *see* religion
Civil Rights Movement 40
collective 10, 13, 15, 42, 44, 51, 70, 74, 84, 91, 97, 108, 110–11, 114, 118, 121, 122, 128, 129, 143, 147, 151, 173, 174, 176, 178, 187, 190, 195, 197, 204, 208, 233, 234–35; consciousness 75, 145; power 9, 18, 198, 218; groups as 124, 155, 166, 192, 238, 240; *see also* The Spiral Goddess Collective

Collins, Patricia Hill 170; *see also Black Feminist Thought*
colonization 39, 40, 94, 95, 108, 180; *see also* decolonization
Combahee River Collective 166, 240
community xii, 11, 16, 18, 29, 31, 38, 43, 58, 75, 85, 102, 105, 106, 108, 109, 111, 127, 142, 144, 148, 160, 161, 171, 186–87, 188, 223, 225, 227, 231; local 81, 116–117, 120–1, 141–2, 192–94, 231, 233, 235, 236; the yoga community 8, 14, 201
consciousness 8, 43, 58, 88, 91, 92, 104, 108, 170, 184; collective 75, 145; consciousness-raising 13, 188 ; critical 7, 68, 84, 99, 105, 109, 148, 164, 195, 196, 198, 231, 238; global 135; oppositional 165; popular 235; radical 99; universal 57, 61; *see also* woke
Cooper, Brittany 124; *see also* Crunk Feminist Collective
Covid-19 13–14, 20, 132, 135, 170, 195, 221; *see also* pandemic
Crenshaw, Kimberlé 166–67
Crunk Feminist Collective 124; *see also* Cooper, Brittany
cultural appropriation 2, 8, 11–12, 15, 86, 88–89, 94, 103, 160, 164, 167, 169, 235
cultural criticism 16, 68–69, 149, 165–66, 236; critical theory 68, cultural studies 9; *see also* women's studies

dance 5, 31, 84, 94, 133, 136, 185, 191–93, 199, 209–19, 231; *see also* JourneyDance
Davis, Angela 109, 169
decolonization 93, 94, 96; *see also* colonization
The Deepest Well 112, 238; *see also* Harris, Nadine Burke
DEI (Diversity, Equity, and Inclusion) 14, 98–99; *see also* diversity
Denmark 59, 77, 78, 79, 140, 212
depression 35, 45, 55, 81, 157, 181, 238, 240; *see also* anxiety; mental health
disability 17, 71, 74, 118–122, 148, 239, 241; *see also* ableism
Disability Justice Movement 17, 122
Disability Visibility 119, 241; *see also* Wong, Alice
diversity 15, 68, 91–94, 97, 99, 165; *see also* DEI

EFT (Emotional Freedom Technique) 133

Ehrenreich, Barbara 70–71, 238; see also *Natural Causes*
Embodied Self-Awakening 75, 180, 238; see also Gesell, Nityda
Embodied Social Justice 56, 103, 127, 143, 191, 214, 231, 238; see also social justice
embodiment 9, 19, 86, 104, 110, 179, 183–85, 194, 199, 123, 235, 238; embodied movement 15, 31, 84, 107, 110, 142, 195, 206, 212, 214, 227, 231, 233–36; embodied yoga 183; see also embodied social justice
The Embody Lab 179, 184, 213, 238; see also Chatterjee, Ananya; williams, the Rev. angel Kyodo
Embrace Yoga's Roots 15, 39, 92, 97, 237; see also Barkataki, Susanna
Emergent Strategy 145, 172, 238–39; see also brown, adrienne maree
Emerson and Hopper 75, 238; see also *Overcoming Trauma Through Yoga*
empaths 148–50, 229
empathy 49, 52, 84, 87, 117, 146, 148–49, 151, 153, 158, 172, 191, 202
empowerment 9, 21, 23, 71, 100, 104, 124, 151, 163, 183, 194, 209, 226
Evans, Stephanie Y. 170–71, 238; see also *Black Women's Yoga History*
Every Body Yoga 38, 120, 168, 240; see also Stanley, Jessamyn

Felon: Poems 208; see also Betts, Reginald Dwayne
feminism 18, 100, 161–3, 164–5, 167, 225–26, 236; Black feminism 164–68, 168–71, 174, 240
Feminist Theory from Margin to Center 165, 240; see also hooks, bell
fitness 5, 8, 10, 16, 18, 29–31, 35, 44, 68–69, 73, 86, 90–91, 97, 105, 108, 116–17, 152, 191, 199, 202, 209–10, 212, 214, 221, 225–27, 234, 236; industry 8, 31; see also *Women and Fitness in American Culture*; workout
flexibility 11, 33, 44, 72, 73, 77, 156, 179, 180, 201–2, 208, 227
Floyd, George 13–14
Forbes, Bo 51, 125, 130–31, 138, 149, 158–59, 176–77, 229, 238; see also *Yoga for Emotional Balance*
freedom 110, 115, 133, 195–98, 199, 208, 210, 214, 216, 217, 218, 224, 239
The Future Is Disabled 121, 239; see also Piepzna-Samarasinha, Leah Lakshmi

Gadsby, Hannah 116; see also *Nanette*
Gay, Roxane 162; see also *Bad Feminist*
gender 17, 52, 66, 67, 91, 107, 108, 112, 117, 154, 161, 164, 169, 206; cisgender 17, 34, 86, 96, 98, 101; fluid/genderqueer, non-binary/non-conforming 74, 101, 148; neutral 201; trans 101, 162
Gesell, Nityda 75, 80, 112, 180, 184, 230, 238; see also *Embodied Self-Awakening*
Girls on Fire 165, 193, 240
gratitude ix, 27, 93, 142
Gumbs, Alexis Pauline 173–74, 213, 238; see also *Undrowned*

Haines, Staci K. 103–4, 111, 128, 144, 238; see also *The Politics of Trauma*
Hamer, Fannie Lou 196
Hapi, Dr. Asar 95
Harris, Nadine Burke 112–14, 238; see also *The Deepest Well*
healing vi, 12, 60, 63, 68, 75, 76, 79, 80–81, 84–85, 103, 108–112, 118, 133, 134, 142, 143, 147–48, 151, 159, 167, 169, 170, 176, 179, 181, 206, 209, 210, 228, 231, 238, 240, 241; breath as 24, 76, 144; integrative 44, 74, 98, 208; modality 85, 88, 133, 154, 163, 191, 192, 194–95, 215–16; narratives 58; physical 44, 97, 114, 122, 132, 158; and transformation 3, 95, 114, 118, 163, 230, 234, 235
The Healing Power of the Breath 24, 144, 238; see also Brown and Gerbarg
healthcare 106, 132, 183
heart-rate variability (HRV) 28
Hersey, Tricia 57, 82, 175–76, 238; see also The Nap Ministry; *Rest Is Resistance*
Heyman, Jivana 14–15, 41–42, 93, 109, 118–20, 188–89, 233, 235, 240; see also *Accessible Yoga*; *Yoga Revolution*
Hobart and Kneese 109, 127–29, 239
Holding Change vi, 172, 238; see also brown, adrienne maree
hooks, bell 15, 18, 68, 99, 149, 164, 166, 238, 239, 240; see also *Feminist Theory from Margin to Center*; *Talking About a Revolution*
Horton, Carol 42, 163, 239, 240; see also *21st Century Yoga*; *Yoga Ph.D.*
Horton and Harvey 42, 240; see also *21st Century Yoga*
Hotep, Yirser Ra 95, 239; see also Kemetic Yoga

Howard, Leslie 182, 239; *see also Pelvic Liberation*
Huberman, Andrew 122
imagination 26, 59, 65, 108, 144–46, 148, 150, 153, 154, 157, 167, 171–72, 175, 187
imperialism 8, 18, 82, 148
In the Realm of Hungry Ghosts 106, 241; *see also* Maté, Dr. Gabor
India xii, 7, 39–40, 87, 88–9, 90, 92, 93–94, 95, 171, 179, 196, 204, 237–38
indigenous 7, 8, 87, 89, 92, 130, 141, 190
Insight Timer 56
interdisciplinary 9, 15, 105, 166; transdisciplinary 9, 18, 230; *see also* academia
intersectionality xiii, 17, 86, 92–3, 97, 117, 119, 163, 165–66, 167, 191

Johnson, Michelle Cassandra vi, 13–15, 34, 73, 97–99, 169, 230, 239; *see also Skill in Action*
JourneyDance ix, 16, 31, 61–62, 103, 131, 135, 163, 192, 214–15, 231, 236; *see also* dance

Kegels 181–82
Kemetic Yoga 95, 238, 239; *see also* Hotep, Yirser Ra; yoga
Kim and Schalk 127–28, 239
Kingston, Maxine Hong 152–53, 239; *see also The Woman Warrior*
Kipp, Eric 140
Kundalini yoga 101, 102, 108; *see also* yoga

Lasater, Judith 40–43, 57, 186, 197, 239; *see also Living Your Yoga*
Law, Naomi 196, 239
LeGuin, Ursula xii
Levine, Peter 75, 241; *see also Waking the Tiger*
LGBTQIA+ 117, 161; *see also* queer
Liberated to the Bone vi, 10, 230; *see also* Raffo, Susan
Liberation Institute 189
Living Your Yoga 40, 43, 57, 186, 197, 239; *see also* Lasater, Judith
Long, Jana 170, 239; *see also The Uncommon Yogi*
Lorde, Audre 124, 171, 239; *see also A Burst of Light*
love vi, xii–xiii, 12, 23, 27, 29, 41, 49, 52, 57, 59, 60, 66, 69, 80, 115, 116, 142, 144, 154, 158, 186, 191, 194, 202, 204, 207, 228, 232; self-love xii–xiii, 52, 124, 126–27, 132; warriors 147–48, 151, 239

Maine 116, 140, 189, 192, 221, 231
Maine State Prison system 189
mainstream *see* American
mantras 36, 41, 56, 57–59, 136
Marich, Jamie vi, 76, 219, 239; *see also Process Not Perfection*
massage 130–31, 132–33, 159–60
Maté, Dr. Gabor 106, 241; *see also In the Realm of Hungry Ghosts*
meditation 1, 9, 18, 19, 38, 39, 49, 55–57, 58, 59, 60, 71, 84, 108, 110, 120, 129, 134, 135, 136, 169, 170, 172, 173–74, 179, 184, 187, 188, 193, 208, 209, 215, 241; *see also* monkey mind; yoga
Menakem, Resmaa 4, 76, 82, 113, 158–59, 169, 234–35, 239; *see also My Grandmother's Hands*
mental health 11, 49, 110, 113, 158, 171, 182 ; therapy 61, 127; *see also* anxiety; depression
#MeToo Movement 79
microaggressions 34
Middle East 70, 152
Monáe, Janelle 118, 135, 138, 217–18
monkey mind 18, 56, 124; *see also* meditation
Mudras for Modern Life 129, 241; *see also* Saradananda, Swami
My Grandmother's Hands 4, 76, 169, 239; *see also* Menakem, Resmaa
Myers, Nikki 108; *see also* Yoga of Twelve-Step Recovery (Y12SR)

Naboso Neuro Ball 131
namaste 88, 232
Nanette 116; *see also* Gadsby, Hannah
The Nap Ministry 175; *see also* Hersey, Tricia
National Women's Studies Association (NWSA) 124, 163, 169, 239; *see also* Thompson, Becky
Natural Causes 71, 238; *see also* Ehrenreich, Barbara
neuroscience 179, 229; *see also* science
New York 101, 140, 217, 218
non-violence *see* violence
nursing 44, 45, 74, 98, 208, 219, 230

oppression 7, 8, 10, 17, 42, 49, 67, 70, 73, 91, 92, 98, 108, 109, 116, 125, 144,

161, 166, 168, 169, 184, 188–89, 190–91, 197, 215; *see also* privilege; racism; white supremacy
oracle cards 61–4
Orloff, Judith 147–48, 156, 239; *see also Thriving as an Empath*
Overcoming Trauma Through Yoga 75, 238; *see also* Emerson and Hopper
Ozeki, Ruth 179

pandemic 13, 14, 80, 111, 170, 195; *see also* Covid-19
Pandemic of Love 186–7; *see also* Tygielski, Shelly
parasympathetic nervous system 24, 81, 131, 158, 178; *see also* vagus nerve
Parker, Gail 15, 34, 58, 76, 84, 104, 113–15, 136, 175, 176, 178, 184, 185, 198, 230, 232, 239; *see also Restorative Yoga for Ethnic and Race-Based Stress and Trauma*; *Transforming Ethnic and Race-Based Traumatic Stress with Yoga*
Patanjali 41, 167, 240; *see also Yoga Sutras*
patriarchy 18, 88, 143, 162, 164–67, 180, 191, 226
pelvic floor 25, 129, 180–83
Pelvic Liberation 182, 239; *see also* Howard, Leslie
people of color *see* BIPOC
perfectionism 10, 36, 82, 129, 150
personality 53–55
philosophy 7, 33, 39, 41, 42, 43, 48, 95, 135, 146, 167, 172, 179, 204
Piepzna-Samarasinha, Leah Lakshmi 119, 120, 148, 239; *see also Care Work*; *The Future Is Disabled*
Pleasure Activism 17, 172, 185, 238; *see also* brown, adrienne maree
poetry 171, 200, 207–8, 211–12, 225; anatomy as 46, 225
politics 12, 40, 94, 99, 127–28, 166, 190; identity 15, 196; left and right 12, 16, 49, 52, 99 172, 186–87, 196
The Politics of Trauma 103, 111, 238; *see also* Haines, Staci K.
Porges, Stephen 159
positive thinking 49, 57, 69–70, 107
pranayama 24, 38; bee's breath 23, 25, 141, 224; belly breathing 25–26, 159; equal ratio 23, 26; heart-centered 27–28; horse lips 223; paradoxical 26; three-part 25; *ujjayi* 24; *see also* breath

privilege 2, 10, 12, 14, 16–17, 34, 48–49, 67–68, 73, 84–87, 90, 92, 94, 95, 97, 98, 108, 119, 125, 130, 136, 137, 155, 161, 164, 187, 188–89, 190–91, 193, 195; *see also* oppression
Process Not Perfection vi, 76, 219, 239; *see also* Marich, Jamie
Prodependence 37, 241; *see also* Weiss, Robert
pronouns 12, 16, 17, 201
psychology 53–54, 76, 156, 160
PTSD (Post-Traumatic Stress Disorder) 12, 45, 75, 79, 107, 147, 167, 183

queer 17, 52, 63, 101, 108, 115–18, 122, 130, 148, 172, 174, 231, 234; *see also* LGBTQIA+
A Queer Dharma 15, 40, 69, 109, 180, 237; *see also* Ballard, Jacoby
Queer Yoga Youth Project 116

racism 8, 13, 15, 70, 82, 98, 111, 114, 169, 240; *see also* oppression; white supremacy
Raffo, Susan vi, 10, 12, 45–6, 88, 91, 109, 110, 128, 133, 150–51, 159, 200, 225, 239; *see also Liberated to the Bone*
Reagan, Ronald 196
Recovery 2.0 108, 241; *see also* Rosen, Tommy
Reiki 102, 132, 154
religion 9, 16, 33, 66, 100, 103, 179, 234; Christianity 62, 103; *see also* spirituality
resilience 22, 85, 103, 145, 170, 188–89, 210
Rest Is Resistance 175–76, 238; *see also* Hersey, Tricia
Restorative Yoga for Ethnic and Race-Based Stress and Trauma 15, 104, 113–14, 136, 175, 178, 184, 239; *see also* Parker, Gail
Roe v. Wade 189, 238
Róisín, Fariha 184, 240; *see also Who Is Wellness For?*
Rosen, Tommy 108, 241; *see also Recovery 2.0*

The Salt Eaters 216, 237; *see also* Bambara, Toni Cade
Sanskrit 2, 35, 38, 57, 96
Saradananda, Swami 129, 241; *see also Mudras for Modern Life*
savasana (final relaxation) 44, 53, 173, 174, 176, 197, 231–32, 224

Schwartz, Arielle 76, 110–11, 159, 240; see also *Therapeutic Yoga for Trauma Recovery*
science 27–28, 41, 45–46, 54, 69, 70, 76, 80, 135, 157, 158, 172, 181, 215, 241; science fiction 146, 154, 174; see also neuroscience
Science of Yoga 46, 241; see also Swanson, Ann
Sea Change Yoga ix-x, 132, 189, 238; see also Boyson, Elise
self-care 7, 30, 44, 63, 109, 120, 124–29, 163, 168, 169–70, 171, 176, 186–87, 221, 239, 240; see also care
self-study (*svādhyāya*) 15, 19, 30, 42, 46–8, 156, 178, 229, 231, 237
Set Boundaries, Find Peace 125, 240; see also Tawwab, Nedra Glover
sex 17, 37, 60, 61, 78, 106, 107, 132; sexism 23, 165, 166, 206; sexual violence and trauma 77–80, 97, 13, 182, 240; sexuality 9, 17, 66, 67, 91, 115, 152, 154, 163, 165
Shaw, Beth ix, 230; see also YogaFit
Sit Down to Rise Up 186, 240; see also Tygielski, Shelly
Skill in Action 13, 14, 73, 97, 239; see also Johnson, Michelle Cassandra
social justice vi, xii, 8, 11–12, 15, 34, 63, 75, 83, 84, 86–7, 92–3, 94, 96, 97–8, 103, 109–11, 117, 124, 128, 147, 151, 162, 163, 165, 168, 169, 172, 179, 185, 187–89, 190–91, 193, 201, 225, 231, 236, 238, 240; see also Embodied Social Justice
social media 1, 10, 11, 12, 167, 193, 20, 205, 229
socialization 16, 145
somatics 111, 113, 172, 179, 180, 185, 231, 238
South Asian 40, 87, 92, 93–94, 96, 196
space xii, 3, 9, 15, 19, 33, 45, 46, 56, 61, 66, 67–68, 88, 96, 98, 121, 124, 129, 130, 151, 153, 156, 164, 174, 180, 183, 191–2, 198, 213, 218; academic 10, 83, 89, 98–99, 163, 165; in the body/mind 25, 38, 56, 67, 68, 105, 129–30, 197, 207, 232; brave/safe 34, 73, 77, 109, 212, 217, 240; community 121, 233, 236; cultural 12, 37, 117, 118, 162, 235; as ether 26–27; fitness 117, 152, 199; holding of 13, 214; (in)accessible 120–21, 122, 141, 193; natural/public 24, 35, 140, 142–43, 206, 215, 236; sacred 110; as social media/online 10,

89, 174, 180, 196, 229; as studio 31, 37, 45, 63, 67, 74, 77, 88, 116, 117, 174, 179, 190, 192–3, 199–200; as universe xii; yoga 10, 11, 12, 15, 29, 31, 34, 37, 38, 42, 47, 56, 66, 69, 73–74, 75, 77, 87, 89, 91, 92, 93, 94, 97, 99, 101, 109–10, 118, 130, 146–47, 151, 152, 153, 179, 190, 196, 217
The Spiral Goddess Collective 31, 63, 64, 74, 116, 118, 121, 142, 191–94; see also collective
spirituality 3, 33, 43, 89, 100, 103–4, 105, 148, 168, 235; see also religion
Stanley, Jessamyn vi, 10–11, 38, 42, 73, 89–90, 96, 120, 168, 230, 240; see also *Every Body Yoga; Yoke*
Swanson, Ann 46, 241; see also *Science of Yoga*

A Tale for the Time Being 179; see also Ozeki, Ruth
Talking About a Revolution 99, 238; see also hooks, bell
Tantric yoga 64, 78; see also yoga
tarot see oracle cards
Tatum, Beverly Daniel 13, 92, 240
Tawwab, Nedra Glover 125, 240; see also *Set Boundaries, Find Peace*
Taylor, Sonya Renee xii-xiii, 115, 127, 166, 200, 240; see also *The Body Is Not an Apology*
teaching 10, 12, 14, 20, 30, 31, 36, 40–2, 57, 68, 73, 74, 78–80, 86–87, 90, 109, 136, 168, 177, 178, 191, 193, 195, 199, 212, 214, 222–23, 226, 233, 235, 236, 240; trauma-informed 74, 109, 117, 230, 231; yoga teachings 40, 41–42, 120; see also academia
Therapeutic Yoga for Trauma Recovery 76, 110, 240; see also Schwartz, Arielle
Thompson, Becky 163, 169; see also NWSA
Thriving as an Empath 147, 239; see also Orloff, Judith
transformation 3, 4, 5, 8, 9, 13, 14, 22, 31, 73, 85, 88, 95, 98, 100, 114, 145, 163, 167, 172, 187, 194, 211, 213, 214, 230, 231, 234; collective 122, 172, 218, 234–35; cultural 199, 225; embodied 104, 185, 200, 226; structural 112, 127, 148, 151, 168; see also change
Transforming Ethnic and Race-Based Traumatic Stress with Yoga 58, 113, 239; see also Parker, Gail

transgender *see* gender
trauma 5, 14–15, 17, 34, 37, 74–81, 103, 105, 106, 108–14, 132, 152, 184, 189, 209, 231, 238–41; and addiction 105, 106, 108; collective 110, 111, 197; cultural 84, 206; highly activated 150–51; in the body 4, 77, 109, 110, 113, 116, 169, 206, 235; intergenerational 110, 113, 152, 181, 235; race-based 15, 58, 76, 113, 114, 169, 230, 234; response 24, 78, 79, 110, 134–35; sexual 77, 79, 80, 182; systemic 144; trauma-informed 77, 80, 109, 116, 117, 121, 189, 193, 230–31
Trauma-Informed Yoga for Survivors of Sexual Assault 80, 240; *see also* Yamasaki, Zahabiyah A.
Treleven, David 77
Trump, Donald 85, 128
21st Century Yoga 42, 240; *see also* Horton, Carol; Horton and Harvey
Tygielski, Shelly 186–87, 240; *see also* Pandemic of Love; *Sit Down to Rise Up*

The Uncommon Yogi 170, 239; *see also* Long, Jana
Undrowned 173, 213, 238; *see also* Gumbs, Alexis Pauline
University of Maine system 14

vagus nerve 131, 158–60; *see also* parasympathetic nervous system
violence 40, 117, 205, 119, 128, 144; non-violence 40–41, 190, 204, 205; patriarchal 85, 163; sexual 76–77

Waking the Tiger 75, 241; *see also* Levine, Peter
warriors 146–48, 217, 148, 153; love 147, 148, 151, 239; poses 129, 140, 152, 210, 223; social justice 98; woman 151–53, 240
Weintraub, Amy 7, 158, 181, 240; *see also Yoga for Depression*
Weis, Robert 37, 241; see also *Prodependence*
West, Cornel 147, 238–39
white supremacy 2, 13, 82–83, 85, 88, 97–98, 114, 125, 128, 137, 143, 150, 162, 169, 190–91, 226; *see also* oppression; racism
Who Is Wellness For? 184, 240; *see also* Róisín, Fariha
Wikipedia 41, 100, 240
williams, the Rev. angel Kyodo 179–80, 183; *see also* The Embody Lab

Wint, Brandon 115
woke 12, 14, 34, 99, 190; *see also* consciousness
The Woman Warrior 152, 239; *see also* Kingston, Maxine Hong
Women and Fitness in American Culture 31, 42, 90, 201, 225, 238; *see also* fitness
women's studies 9, 163; *see also* academia
Wong, Alice 119, 241; *see also Disability Visibility*
workout 32, 33–34, 35, 128, 167, 227; *see also* fitness

Yamasaki, Zahabiyah A. 77, 80, 230, 240–41; *see also Trauma-Informed Yoga for Survivors of Sexual Assault*
Yang, Larry 197
YMCA (Young Men's Christian Association) x, 191, 210, 221, 222, 224
Yoga: eight limbs 38, 48, 96, 111, 235; karma 186; nidra 56, 122, 193; *niyama* 48; personal practice 3, 30, 57, 61, 86, 137, 177; physical practice 8, 33–4, 38–9, 97, 118, 120, 121, 167, 179, 189, 236; restorative 58, 113, 114, 125, 176–78, 215, 229, 239; subtle body 6, 48, 153; *yama* 204; *see also* American yoga; *asanas*; Kemetic yoga; Kundalini yoga; meditation, Tantric yoga
Yoga Alliance 1, 30, 90, 95
Yoga for Depression 181, 240; *see also* Weintraub, Amy
Yoga for Emotional Balance 229, 238; *see also* Forbes, Bo
Yoga for Everyone 120; *see also* Bondy, Dianne
Yoga Journal 41; LIVE! conference 1, 101, 140, 217
Yoga of Twelve-Step Recovery (Y12SR) 108, 240; *see also* Myers, Nikki
Yoga Ph.D. 42, 239; *see also* Horton, Carol
Yoga Revolution 15, 41, 120, 238; *see also* Heyman, Jivana
Yoga Sutras 41, 240; *see also* Patanjali
YogaFit ix, 29, 36, 42, 177, 182, 230–31; *see also* Shaw, Beth
Yoke vi, 10, 38, 42, 89, 230, 240; *see also* Stanley, Jessamyn

Zentangle Method 220, 237
Zoom 61, 121, 132, 135, 147, 163, 174, 180, 213, 221

www.ingramcontent.com/pod-product-compliance
Ingram Content Group UK Ltd.
Pitfield, Milton Keynes, MK11 3LW, UK
UKHW032021300125
454454UK00015B/173

transgender *see* gender
trauma 5, 14–15, 17, 34, 37, 74–81, 103, 105, 106, 108–14, 132, 152, 184, 189, 209, 231, 238–41; and addiction 105, 106, 108; collective 110, 111, 197; cultural 84, 206; highly activated 150–51; in the body 4, 77, 109, 110, 113, 116, 169, 206, 235; intergenerational 110, 113, 152, 181, 235; race-based 15, 58, 76, 113, 114, 169, 230, 234; response 24, 78, 79, 110, 134–35; sexual 77, 79, 80, 182; systemic 144; trauma-informed 77, 80, 109, 116, 117, 121, 189, 193, 230–31
Trauma-Informed Yoga for Survivors of Sexual Assault 80, 240; *see also* Yamasaki, Zahabiyah A.
Treleven, David 77
Trump, Donald 85, 128
21st Century Yoga 42, 240; *see also* Horton, Carol; Horton and Harvey
Tygielski, Shelly 186–87, 240; *see also* Pandemic of Love; *Sit Down to Rise Up*

The Uncommon Yogi 170, 239; *see also* Long, Jana
Undrowned 173, 213, 238; *see also* Gumbs, Alexis Pauline
University of Maine system 14

vagus nerve 131, 158–60; *see also* parasympathetic nervous system
violence 40, 117, 205, 119, 128, 144; non-violence 40–41, 190, 204, 205; patriarchal 85, 163; sexual 76–77

Waking the Tiger 75, 241; *see also* Levine, Peter
warriors 146–48, 217, 148, 153; love 147, 148, 151, 239; poses 129, 140, 152, 210, 223; social justice 98; woman 151–53, 240
Weintraub, Amy 7, 158, 181, 240; *see also Yoga for Depression*
Weis, Robert 37, 241; see also *Prodependence*
West, Cornel 147, 238–39
white supremacy 2, 13, 82–83, 85, 88, 97–98, 114, 125, 128, 137, 143, 150, 162, 169, 190–91, 226; *see also* oppression; racism
Who Is Wellness For? 184, 240; *see also* Róisín, Fariha
Wikipedia 41, 100, 240
williams, the Rev. angel Kyodo 179–80, 183; *see also* The Embody Lab

Wint, Brandon 115
woke 12, 14, 34, 99, 190; *see also* consciousness
The Woman Warrior 152, 239; *see also* Kingston, Maxine Hong
Women and Fitness in American Culture 31, 42, 90, 201, 225, 238; *see also* fitness
women's studies 9, 163; *see also* academia
Wong, Alice 119, 241; *see also Disability Visibility*
workout 32, 33–34, 35, 128, 167, 227; *see also* fitness

Yamasaki, Zahabiyah A. 77, 80, 230, 240–41; *see also Trauma-Informed Yoga for Survivors of Sexual Assault*
Yang, Larry 197
YMCA (Young Men's Christian Association) x, 191, 210, 221, 222, 224
Yoga: eight limbs 38, 48, 96, 111, 235; karma 186; nidra 56, 122, 193; *niyama* 48; personal practice 3, 30, 57, 61, 86, 137, 177; physical practice 8, 33–4, 38–9, 97, 118, 120, 121, 167, 179, 189, 236; restorative 58, 113, 114, 125, 176–78, 215, 229, 239; subtle body 6, 48, 153; *yama* 204; *see also* American yoga; *asanas*; Kemetic yoga; Kundalini yoga; meditation, Tantric yoga
Yoga Alliance 1, 30, 90, 95
Yoga for Depression 181, 240; *see also* Weintraub, Amy
Yoga for Emotional Balance 229, 238; *see also* Forbes, Bo
Yoga for Everyone 120; *see also* Bondy, Dianne
Yoga Journal 41; LIVE! conference 1, 101, 140, 217
Yoga of Twelve-Step Recovery (Y12SR) 108, 240; *see also* Myers, Nikki
Yoga Ph.D. 42, 239; *see also* Horton, Carol
Yoga Revolution 15, 41, 120, 238; *see also* Heyman, Jivana
Yoga Sutras 41, 240; *see also* Patanjali
YogaFit ix, 29, 36, 42, 177, 182, 230–31; *see also* Shaw, Beth
Yoke vi, 10, 38, 42, 89, 230, 240; *see also* Stanley, Jessamyn

Zentangle Method 220, 237
Zoom 61, 121, 132, 135, 147, 163, 174, 180, 213, 221

www.ingramcontent.com/pod-product-compliance
Ingram Content Group UK Ltd.
Pitfield, Milton Keynes, MK11 3LW, UK
UKHW032021300125
454454UK00015B/173